INDIAN COOKBOOK 2022

MOUTH-WATERING RECIPES FROM THE REGIONAL TRADITION

FOR BEGINNERS

EMILIE BUSH

Table of Contents

Vegetable Patties 18
    Ingredients 18
    Method 19
Sprouted Beans Bhel 20
    Ingredients 20
    For the garnish: 20
    Method 21
Aloo Kachori 22
    Ingredients 22
    Method 22
Diet Dosa 23
    Ingredients 23
    Method 23
Nutri Roll 25
    Ingredients 25
    Method 26
Sabudana Palak Doodhi Uttapam 27
    Ingredients 27
    Method 28
Poha 29
    Ingredients 29
    Method 30
Vegetable Cutlet 31

- Ingredients 31
- Method 32
- Soy Bean Uppit 33
  - Ingredients 33
  - Method 34
- Upma 35
  - Ingredients 35
  - Method 36
- Vermicelli Upma 37
  - Ingredients 37
  - Method 38
- Bonda 39
  - Ingredients 39
  - Method 40
- Instant Dhokla 41
  - Ingredients 41
  - Method 42
- Dhal Maharani 43
  - Ingredients 43
  - Method 44
- Milagu Kuzhambu 45
  - Ingredients 45
  - Method 46
- Dhal Hariyali 47
  - Ingredients 47
  - Method 48
- Dhalcha 49

  Ingredients 49

  Method 50

Tarkari Dhalcha 51

  Ingredients 51

  Method 52

Dhokar Dhalna 53

  Ingredients 53

  Method 53

Varan 55

  Ingredients 55

  Method 55

Sweet Dhal 56

  Ingredients 56

  Method 57

Sweet & Sour Dhal 58

  Ingredients 58

  Method 59

Mung-ni-Dhal 60

  Ingredients 60

  Method 61

Dhal with Onion & Coconut 62

  Ingredients 62

  Method 63

Dahi Kadhi 64

  Ingredients 64

  Method 65

Spinach Dhal 66

- Ingredients 66
- Method 67
- Tawker Dhal 68
  - Ingredients 68
  - Method 69
- Basic Dhal 70
  - Ingredients 70
  - Method 71
- Maa-ki-Dhal 72
  - Ingredients 72
  - Method 73
- Dhansak 74
  - Ingredients 74
  - For the dhal mixture: 74
  - Method 75
- Masoor Dhal 76
  - Ingredients 76
  - Method 76
- Panchemel Dhal 77
  - Ingredients 77
  - Method 78
- Cholar Dhal 79
  - Ingredients 79
  - Method 80
- Dilpasand Dhal 81
  - Ingredients 81
  - Method 82

- Dhal Masoor ... 83
  - Ingredients ... 83
  - Method ... 84
- Dhal with Aubergine ... 85
  - Ingredients ... 85
  - Method ... 86
- Yellow Dhal Tadka ... 87
  - Ingredients ... 87
  - Method ... 87
- Rasam ... 88
  - Ingredients ... 88
  - For the spice mixture: ... 88
  - Method ... 89
- Simple Mung Dhal ... 90
  - Ingredients ... 90
  - Method ... 90
- Whole Green Mung ... 91
  - Ingredients ... 91
  - Method ... 92
- Dahi Kadhi with Pakoras ... 93
  - Ingredients ... 93
  - For the kadhi: ... 93
  - Method ... 94
- Sweet Unripe Mango Dhal ... 95
  - Ingredients ... 95
  - Method ... 96
- Malai Dhal ... 97

Ingredients	97
Method	98
Sambhar	99
Ingredients	99
For the seasoning:	99
Method	100
Three Dhals	101
Ingredients	101
Method	102
Methi-Drumstick Sambhar	103
Ingredients	103
Method	104
Dhal Shorba	105
Ingredients	105
Method	105
Yummy Mung	106
Ingredients	106
Method	107
Masala Toor Dhal	108
Ingredients	108
Method	109
Dry Yellow Mung Dhal	110
Ingredients	110
Method	110
Whole Urad	111
Ingredients	111
Method	112

- Dhal Fry 113
  - Ingredients 113
  - Method 114
- Kale Moti ki Biryani 115
  - Ingredients 115
  - Method 116
- Mince & Masoor Pulao 118
  - Ingredients 118
  - Method 119
- Chicken Biryani 120
  - Ingredients 120
  - For the marinade: 120
  - Method 121
- Prawn Biryani 123
  - Ingredients 123
  - For the spice mixture: 123
  - Method 124
- Egg Potato Biryani 125
  - Ingredients 125
  - For the paste: 126
  - Method 126
- Mince Pulao 128
  - Ingredients 128
  - Method 129
- Chana Pulao 130
  - Ingredients 130
  - Method 130

- Simple Khichdi 132
    - Ingredients 132
    - Method 132
- Masala Rice 133
    - Ingredients 133
    - Method 134
- Onion Rice 135
    - Ingredients 135
    - Method 135
- Steamed Rice 137
    - Ingredients 137
    - Method 137
- Stuffed Aubergines 138
    - Ingredients 138
    - Method 138
- Sarson ka Saag 139
    - Ingredients 139
    - Method 140
- Shahi Paneer 141
    - Ingredients 141
    - Method 142
- Tandoori Potato 143
    - Ingredients 143
    - Method 143
- Corn Curry 145
    - Ingredients 145
    - Method 146

Masala Green Pepper 147
    Ingredients 147
    Method 148
No-oil Bottle Gourd 149
    Ingredients 149
    Method 149
Okra with Yoghurt 150
    Ingredients 150
    Method 151
Sautéed Karela 152
    Ingredients 152
    Method 153
Cabbage with Peas 154
    Ingredients 154
    Method 154
Potatoes in Tomato Sauce 155
    Ingredients 155
    Method 155
Matar Palak 156
    Ingredients 156
    Method 157
Masala Cabbage 158
    Ingredients 158
    Method 159
Aubergine Curry 160
    Ingredients 160
    Method 161

Simla Mirch ka Bharta 162
    Ingredients 162
    Method 163
Quick Bottle Gourd Curry 164
    Ingredients 164
    Method 164
Kaala Chana Curry 165
    Ingredients 165
    Method 166
Kalina 167
    Ingredients 167
    Method 168
Tandoori Cauliflower 169
    Ingredients 169
    Method 169
Spicy Kaala Chana 170
    Ingredients 170
    Method 171
Tur Dhal Kofta 172
    Ingredients 172
    Method 172
Shahi Cauliflower 173
    Ingredients 173
    Method 174
Okra Gojju 175
    Ingredients 175
    Method 175

Yam in Green Sauce 176
    Ingredients.. 176
    For the sauce: 176
    Method 177
Simla Mirch ki Sabzi 178
    Ingredients.. 178
    Method 179
Cauliflower Curry 180
    Ingredients.. 180
    Method 180
Haaq 181
    Ingredients.. 181
    Method 182
Dry Cauliflower 183
    Ingredients.. 183
    Method 183
Vegetable Korma 184
    Ingredients.. 184
    Method 185
Fried Aubergine 186
    Ingredients.. 186
    For the marinade: 186
    Method 186
Red Tomato Curry 187
    Ingredients.. 187
    Method 188
Aloo Matar Curry 189

- Ingredients 189
  - Method 190
- Badshahi Baingan 191
  - Ingredients 191
  - Method 192
- Potatoes in Garam Masala 193
  - Ingredients 193
  - Method 193
- Tamilian Korma 194
  - Ingredients 194
  - For the spice mixture: 194
  - Method 195
- Dry Aubergine with Onion & Potato 196
  - Ingredients 196
  - Method 196
- Koftas Lajawab 197
  - Ingredients 197
  - For the koftas: 197
  - Method 198
- Teekha Baingan Masala 199
  - Ingredients 199
  - Method 199
- Vegetable Kofta 200
  - Ingredients 200
  - Method 201
- Dry Pumpkin 202
  - Ingredients 202

- Method 202
- Mixed Vegetables with Fenugreek 203
  - Ingredients 203
  - Method 204
- Dum Gobhi 205
  - Ingredients 205
  - Method 205
- Chhole 206
  - Ingredients 206
  - Method 207
- Aubergine Curry with Onion & Potato 208
  - Ingredients 208
  - Method 209
- Simple Bottle Gourd 210
  - Ingredients 210
  - Method 210
- Mixed Vegetable Curry 211
  - Ingredients 211
  - Method 212
- Dry Mixed Vegetables 213
  - Ingredients 213
  - Method 214
- Dry Potatoes & Peas 215
  - Ingredients 215
  - Method 215
- Dhokar Dhalna 216
  - Ingredients 216

Method 217
Spicy Fried Potatoes 218
　　Ingredients 218
　　Method 218

Vegetable Patties

Makes 12

Ingredients

2 tbsp arrowroot powder

4-5 large potatoes, boiled and grated

1 tbsp refined vegetable oil plus extra for frying

125g/4½oz besan*

25g/scant 1oz fresh coconut, grated

4-5 cashew nuts

3-4 raisins

125g/4½oz frozen peas, boiled

2 tsp dried pomegranate seeds

2 tsp coarsely ground coriander

1 tsp fennel seeds

½ tsp ground black pepper

½ tsp chilli powder

1 tsp amchoor*

½ tsp rock salt

Salt to taste

Method

- Knead together the arrowroot, potatoes and 1 tbsp of oil. Set aside.

- To make the filling, mix the remaining ingredients, except the oil.

- Divide the potato dough into round patties. Place a spoonful of the filling in the centre of each patty. Seal them like a pouch and flatten.

- Heat the remaining oil in a saucepan. Shallow fry the patties over a low heat till golden brown. Serve hot.

Sprouted Beans Bhel

(Savoury Snack with Sprouted Beans)

Serves 4

Ingredients

100g/3½oz sprouted mung beans, boiled

250g/9oz kaala chana*, boiled

3 large potatoes, boiled and chopped

2 large tomatoes, finely chopped

1 medium-sized onion, chopped

Salt to taste

For the garnish:

2 tbsp mint chutney

2 tbsp hot and sweet mango chutney

4-5 tbsp yoghurt

100g/3½ oz potato crisps, crushed

10g/¼oz coriander leaves, chopped

Method
- Mix all the ingredients together, except the garnish ingredients.
- Garnish in the order that the ingredients are listed. Serve immediately.

Aloo Kachori

(Fried Potato Dumpling)

Makes 15

Ingredients

350g/12oz wholemeal flour

1 tbsp refined vegetable oil plus extra for deep frying

1 tsp ajowan seeds

Salt to taste

5 potatoes, boiled and mashed

2 tsp chilli powder

1 tbsp coriander leaves, chopped

Method

- Knead the flour, 1 tbsp oil, ajowan seeds and salt together. Divide into lime-sized balls. Flatten each between your palms and set aside.
- Mix together the potatoes, chilli powder, coriander leaves and some salt.
- Place a portion of this mixture in the centre of each patty. Seal by pinching the edges together.
- Heat the oil in a frying pan. Deep fry the kachoris on a medium heat till golden brown. Drain and serve hot.

Diet Dosa

(Diet Crêpe)

Makes 12

Ingredients

300g/10oz mung dhal*, soaked in 250ml/8fl oz water for 3-4 hours

3-4 green chillies

2.5cm/1in root ginger

100g/3½oz semolina

1 tbsp sour cream

50g/1¾oz coriander leaves, chopped

6 curry leaves

Refined vegetable oil for greasing

Salt to taste

Method

- Mix the dhal with the green chillies and ginger. Grind together.
- Add the semolina and sour cream. Mix well. Add the coriander leaves, curry leaves and enough water to make a thick batter.

- Grease a flat pan and heat it. Pour 2 tbsp batter on it and spread with the back of a spoon. Cook for 3 minutes on a low heat. Flip and repeat.
- Repeat for the remaining batter. Serve hot.

Nutri Roll

Makes 8-10

Ingredients

200g/7oz spinach, finely chopped

1 carrot, finely chopped

125g/4½oz frozen peas

50g/1¾oz sprouted mung beans

3-4 large potatoes, boiled and mashed

2 large onions, finely chopped

½ tsp ginger paste

½ tsp garlic paste

1 green chilli, finely chopped

½ tsp amchoor*

Salt to taste

½ tsp chilli powder

3 tbsp coriander leaves, finely chopped

Refined vegetable oil for shallow frying

8-10 chapattis

2 tbsp hot and sweet mango chutney

Method

- Steam the spinach, carrots, peas and mung beans together.
- Mix the steamed vegetables with the potatoes, onions, ginger paste, garlic paste, green chilli, amchoor, salt, chilli powder and coriander leaves. Knead well to make a smooth mixture.
- Shape the mixture into small cutlets.
- Heat the oil in a saucepan. Shallow fry the cutlets on a medium heat till golden brown. Drain and set aside.
- Spread some hot and sweet mango chutney over a chapatti. Place a cutlet in the centre and roll the chapatti up.
- Repeat for all the chapattis. Serve hot.

Sabudana Palak Doodhi Uttapam

(Sago, Spinach and Bottle Gourd Pancake)

Makes 20

Ingredients

1 tsp toor dhal*

1 tsp mung dhal*

1 tsp urad beans*

1 tsp masoor dhal*

3 tsp rice

100g/3½ oz sago, coarsely ground

50g/1¾oz spinach, steamed and ground

¼ bottle gourd*, grated

125g/4½oz besan*

½ tsp ground cumin

1 tsp mint leaves, finely chopped

1 green chilli, finely chopped

½ tsp ginger paste

Salt to taste

100ml/3½fl oz water

Refined vegetable oil for frying

Method

- Grind together the toor dhal, mung dhal, urad beans, masoor dhal and rice. Set aside.
- Soak the sago for 3-5 minutes. Drain completely.
- Mix with the ground dhal-and-rice mixture.
- Add the spinach, bottle gourd, besan, ground cumin, mint leaves, green chilli, ginger paste, salt and enough water to make a thick batter. Set aside for 30 minutes.
- Grease a frying pan and heat it. Pour 1 tbsp batter in the pan and spread it with the back of a spoon.
- Cover and cook on a medium heat till the underside is light brown. Flip and repeat.
- Repeat for the remaining batter. Serve hot with tomato ketchup or green coconut chutney

Poha

Serves 4

Ingredients

150g/5½oz poha*

1½ tbsp refined vegetable oil

½ tsp cumin seeds

½ tsp mustard seeds

1 large potato, finely chopped

2 large onions, finely sliced

5-6 green chillies, finely chopped

8 curry leaves, roughly chopped

¼ tsp turmeric

45g/1½oz roasted peanuts (optional)

25g/scant 1oz fresh coconut, grated or scraped

10g/¼oz coriander leaves, finely chopped

1 tsp lemon juice

Salt to taste

Method

- Wash the poha well. Drain the water completely and set the poha aside in a colander for 15 minutes.
- Gently loosen the poha lumps with your fingers. Set aside.
- Heat the oil in a saucepan. Add the cumin and mustard seeds. Let them splutter for 15 seconds.
- Add the chopped potatoes. Stir-fry on a medium heat for 2-3 minutes. Add the onions, green chillies, curry leaves and turmeric. Cook till the onions are translucent. Remove from the heat.
- Add the poha, roasted peanuts and half of the grated coconut and coriander leaves. Toss to mix thoroughly.
- Sprinkle the lemon juice and salt. Cook on a low heat for 4-5 minutes.
- Garnish with the remaining coconut and coriander leaves. Serve hot.

Vegetable Cutlet

Makes 10-12

Ingredients

2 onions, finely chopped

5 garlic cloves

¼ tsp fennel seeds

2-3 green chillies

10g/¼oz coriander leaves, finely chopped

2 large carrots, finely chopped

1 large potato, finely chopped

1 small beetroot, finely chopped

50g/1¾oz French beans, finely chopped

50g/1¾oz green peas

900ml/1½ pints water

Salt to taste

¼ tsp turmeric

2-3 tbsp besan*

1 tbsp refined vegetable oil plus extra for deep frying

50g/1¾oz breadcrumbs

Method

- Grind 1 onion, the garlic, fennel seeds, green chillies and coriander leaves together into a smooth paste. Set aside.
- Mix the carrots, potato, beetroot, French beans and peas together in a saucepan. Add 500ml/16fl oz water, salt and turmeric and cook on a medium heat till the vegetables are soft.
- Mash the vegetables thoroughly and set aside.
- Mix the besan and the remaining water together to form a smooth batter. Set aside.
- Heat 1 tbsp oil in a saucepan. Add the remaining onion and fry till translucent.
- Add the onion-garlic paste and fry for a minute on a medium heat, stirring continuously.
- Add the mashed vegetables and mix thoroughly.
- Remove from the heat and set aside to cool.
- Divide this mixture into 10-12 balls. Flatten between your palms to make patties.
- Dip the patties in the batter and roll in the breadcrumbs.
- Heat the oil in a frying pan. Shallow fry the patties till golden brown on both sides.
- Serve hot with ketchup.

Soy Bean Uppit

(Soy Bean Snack)

Serves 4

Ingredients

1½ tbsp refined vegetable oil

½ tsp mustard seeds

2 green chillies, finely chopped

2 red chillies, finely chopped

Pinch of asafoetida

1 large onion, finely chopped

2.5cm/1in root ginger, julienned

10 garlic cloves, finely chopped

6 curry leaves

100g/3½oz soy bean semolina*, dry roasted

100g/3½oz semolina, dry roasted

200g/7oz peas

500ml/16fl oz hot water

¼ tsp turmeric

1 tsp sugar

1 tsp salt

1 large tomato, finely chopped

2 tbsp coriander leaves, finely chopped

15 raisins

10 cashew nuts

Method

- Heat the oil in a saucepan. Add the mustard seeds. Let them splutter for 15 seconds.
- Add the green chillies, red chillies, asafoetida, onion, ginger, garlic and curry leaves. Fry on a medium heat for 3-4 minutes, stirring frequently.
- Add the soy bean semolina, semolina and the peas. Cook till both the kinds of the semolina turn golden brown.
- Add the hot water, turmeric, sugar and salt. Cook over a medium heat till the water dries up.
- Garnish with the tomato, coriander leaves, raisins and cashew nuts.
- Serve hot.

Upma

(Semolina Breakfast Dish)

Serves 4

Ingredients

1 tbsp ghee

150g/5½oz semolina

1 tbsp refined vegetable oil

¼ tsp mustard seeds

1 tsp urad dhal*

3 green chillies, slit lengthways

8-10 curry leaves

1 medium-sized onion, finely chopped

1 medium-sized tomato, finely chopped

750ml/1¼ pints water

1 heaped tsp sugar

Salt to taste

50g/1¾oz canned peas (optional)

25g/scant 1oz coriander leaves, finely chopped

Method

- Heat the ghee in a frying pan. Add the semolina and fry, stirring frequently, till the semolina turns golden brown. Set aside.
- Heat the oil in a saucepan. Add the mustard seeds, urad dhal, green chillies and curry leaves. Fry till the urad dhal turns brown.
- Add the onion and fry on a low heat till translucent. Add the tomato and fry for another 3-4 minutes.
- Add the water and mix well. Cook on a medium heat till the mixture starts boiling. Stir well.
- Add the sugar, salt, semolina and peas. Mix well.
- Cook on a low heat, stirring continuously for 2-3 minutes.
- Garnish with the coriander leaves. Serve hot.

Vermicelli Upma

(Vermicelli with Onion)

Serves 4

Ingredients

3 tbsp refined vegetable oil

1 tsp mung dhal*

1 tsp urad dhal*

¼ tsp mustard seeds

8 curry leaves

10 peanuts

10 cashew nuts

1 medium potato, finely chopped

1 large carrot, finely chopped

2 green chillies, finely chopped

1cm/½ in root ginger, finely chopped

1 large onion, finely chopped

1 tomato, finely chopped

50g/1¾oz frozen peas

Salt to taste

1 litre/1¾ pints water

200g/7oz vermicelli

2 tbsp ghee

Method

- Heat the oil in a saucepan. Add the mung dhal, urad dhal, mustard seeds and curry leaves. Let them splutter for 30 seconds.
- Add the peanuts and cashew nuts. Fry on a medium heat till golden brown.
- Add the potato and carrot. Fry for 4-5 minutes.
- Add the chillies, ginger, onion, tomato, peas and salt. Cook on a medium heat, stirring frequently, till the vegetables are tender.
- Add the water and bring to a boil. Stir well.
- Add the vermicelli while stirring continuously to make sure no lumps are formed.
- Cover with a lid and cook on a low heat for 5-6 minutes.
- Add the ghee and mix well. Serve hot.

Bonda

(Potato Chop)

Makes 10

Ingredients

5 tbsp refined vegetable oil plus extra for deep frying

½ tsp mustard seeds

2.5mm/1in root ginger, finely chopped

2 green chillies, finely chopped

50g/1¾oz coriander leaves, finely chopped

1 large onion, finely chopped

4 medium-sized potatoes, boiled and mashed

1 large carrot, finely chopped and boiled

125g/4½oz canned peas

Pinch of turmeric

Salt to taste

1 tsp lemon juice

250g/9oz besan*

200ml/7fl oz water

½ tsp baking powder

Method

- Heat 4 tbsp oil in a saucepan. Add the mustard seeds, ginger, green chillies, coriander leaves and onion. Fry on a medium heat, stirring occasionally, till the onion turns brown.
- Add the potatoes, carrot, peas, turmeric and salt. Cook on a low heat for 5-6 minutes, stirring occasionally.
- Sprinkle lemon juice and divide the mixture into 10 balls. Set aside.
- Mix the the besan, water and baking powder with 1 tbsp oil to make the batter.
- Heat the oil in a saucepan. Dip each potato ball in the batter and deep fry on a medium heat till golden brown.
- Serve hot.

Instant Dhokla

(Instant Steamed Savoury Cake)

Makes 15-20

Ingredients

250g/9oz besan*

1 tsp salt

2 tbsp sugar

2 tbsp refined vegetable oil

½ tbsp lemon juice

240ml/8fl oz water

1 tbsp baking powder

1 tsp mustard seeds

2 green chillies, slit lengthways

A few curry leaves

1 tbsp water

2 tbsp coriander leaves, finely chopped

1 tbsp fresh coconut, grated

Method

- Mix together the besan, salt, sugar, 1 tbsp oil, lemon juice and water to make a smooth batter.
- Grease a 20cm/8in round cake tin.
- Add the baking powder to the batter. Mix well and pour immediately in the greased tin. Steam for 20 minutes.
- Pierce with a fork to check if done. If the fork does not come out clean, steam again for 5-10 minutes. Set aside.
- Heat the remaining oil in a saucepan. Add the mustard seeds. Let them splutter for 15 seconds.
- Add the green chillies, curry leaves and water. Cook on a low heat for 2 minutes.
- Pour this mixture over the dhokla and allow it to soak up the liquid.
- Garnish with the coriander leaves and grated coconut.
- Cut into squares and serve with mint chutney

Dhal Maharani

(Black Lentils and Kidney Beans)

Serves 4

Ingredients

150g/5½oz urad dhal*

2 tbsp kidney beans

1.4 litres/2½ pints water

Salt to taste

1 tbsp refined vegetable oil

½ tsp cumin seeds

1 large onion, finely chopped

3 medium-sized tomatoes, chopped

1 tsp ginger paste

½ tsp garlic paste

½ tsp chilli powder

½ tsp garam masala

120ml/4fl oz fresh single cream

Method

- Soak the urad dhal and kidney beans together overnight. Drain and cook together in a saucepan with the water and salt for 1 hour on a medium heat. Set aside.
- Heat the oil in a saucepan. Add the cumin seeds. Let them splutter for 15 seconds.
- Add the onion and fry on a medium heat till golden brown.
- Add the tomatoes. Mix well. Add the ginger paste and garlic paste. Fry for 5 minutes.
- Add the cooked dhal and beans mixture, chilli powder and garam masala. Mix well.
- Add the cream. Simmer for 5 minutes, stirring frequently.
- Serve hot with naan or steamed rice

Milagu Kuzhambu

(Split Red Gram in a Pepper Sauce)

Serves 4

Ingredients

2 tsp ghee

2 tsp coriander seeds

1 tbsp tamarind paste

1 tsp ground black pepper

¼ tsp asafoetida

Salt to taste

1 tbsp toor dhal*, cooked

1 litre/1¾ pints water

¼ tsp mustard seeds

1 green chilli, chopped

¼ tsp turmeric

10 curry leaves

Method

- Heat a few drops of ghee in a saucepan. Add the coriander seeds and fry on a medium heat for 2 minutes. Cool and grind.
- Mix with the tamarind paste, pepper, asafoetida, salt and dhal in a large saucepan.
- Add the water. Mix well and bring to a boil on a medium heat. Set aside.
- Heat the remaining ghee in a saucepan. Add the mustard seeds, green chilli, turmeric and curry leaves. Let them splutter for 15 seconds.
- Add this to the dhal. Serve hot.

Dhal Hariyali

(Leafy Vegetables with Split Bengal Gram)

Serves 4

Ingredients

300g/10oz toor dhal*

1.4 litres/2½ pints water

Salt to taste

2 tbsp ghee

1 tsp cumin seeds

1 onion, finely chopped

½ tsp ginger paste

½ tsp garlic paste

½ tsp turmeric

50g/1¾oz spinach, chopped

10g/¼oz fenugreek leaves, finely chopped

25g/scant 1oz coriander leaves

Method

- Cook the dhal with the water and salt in a saucepan for 45 minutes, stirring frequently. Set aside.
- Heat the ghee in a saucepan. Add the cumin seeds, onion, ginger paste, garlic paste and turmeric. Fry for 2 minutes on a low heat, stirring continuously.
- Add the spinach, fenugreek leaves and the coriander leaves. Mix well and simmer for 5-7 minutes.
- Serve hot with steamed rice

Dhalcha

(Split Bengal Gram with Lamb)

Serves 4

Ingredients

150g/5½oz chana dhal*

150g/5½oz toor dhal*

2.8 litres/5 pints water

Salt to taste

2 tbsp tamarind paste

2 tbsp refined vegetable oil

4 large onions, chopped

5cm/2in root ginger, grated

10 garlic cloves, pounded

750g/1lb 10oz lamb, chopped

1.4 litres/2½ pints water

3-4 tomatoes, chopped

1 tsp chilli powder

1 tsp turmeric

1 tsp garam masala

20 curry leaves

25g/scant 1oz coriander leaves, finely chopped

Method

- Cook the dhals with the water and salt for 1 hour on a medium heat. Add the tamarind paste and mash well. Set aside.
- Heat the oil in a saucepan. Add the onions, ginger and garlic. Fry on a medium heat till brown. Add the lamb and stir constantly till brown.
- Add water and simmer till the lamb is tender.
- Add the tomatoes, chilli powder, turmeric and salt. Mix well. Cook for another 7 minutes.
- Add the dhal, garam masala and curry leaves. Mix well. Simmer for 4-5 minutes.
- Garnish with the coriander leaves. Serve hot.

Tarkari Dhalcha

(Split Bengal Gram with Vegetables)

Serves 4

Ingredients

150g/5½oz chana dhal*

150g/5½oz toor dhal*

Salt to taste

3 litres/5¼ pints water

10g/¼oz mint leaves

10g/¼oz coriander leaves

2 tbsp refined vegetable oil

½ tsp mustard seeds

½ tsp cumin seeds

Pinch of fenugreek seeds

Pinch of kalonji seeds*

2 dry red chillies

10 curry leaves

½ tsp ginger paste

½ tsp garlic paste

½ tsp turmeric

1 tsp chilli powder

1 tsp tamarind paste

500g/1lb 2oz pumpkin, finely diced

Method

- Cook both the dhals with the salt, 2.5 litres/4 pints of water and half the mint and coriander in a saucepan on a medium heat for 1 hour. Grind into a thick paste. Set aside.
- Heat the oil in a saucepan. Add the mustard, cumin, fenugreek and kalonji seeds. Let them splutter for 15 seconds.
- Add the red chillies and curry leaves. Fry on a medium heat for 15 seconds.
- Add the dhal paste, ginger paste, garlic paste, turmeric, chilli powder and tamarind paste. Mix well. Cook on a medium heat, stirring frequently, for 10 minutes.
- Add the remaining water and the pumpkin. Simmer till the pumpkin is cooked.
- Add the remaining mint and coriander leaves. Cook for 3-4 minutes.
- Serve hot.

Dhokar Dhalna

(Fried Dhal Cubes in Curry)

Serves 4

Ingredients

600g/1lb 5oz chana dhal*, soaked overnight

120ml/4fl oz water

Salt to taste

4 tbsp refined vegetable oil plus extra for deep frying

3 green chillies, chopped

½ tsp asafoetida

2 large onions, finely chopped

1 bay leaf

1 tsp ginger paste

1 tsp garlic paste

1 tsp chilli powder

¾ tsp turmeric

1 tsp garam masala

1 tbsp coriander leaves, finely chopped

Method

- Grind the dhal with the water and some salt to a thick paste. Set aside.
- Heat 1 tbsp oil in a saucepan. Add the green chillies and asafoetida. Let them splutter for 15 seconds. Stir in the dhal paste and some more salt. Mix well.
- Spread this mixture on a tray to cool. Cut into 2.5cm/1in pieces.
- Heat the oil for deep frying in a saucepan. Fry the pieces till golden brown. Set aside.
- Heat 2 tbsp oil in a saucepan. Fry the onions till brown. Grind them to a paste and set aside.
- Heat the remaining 1 tbsp oil in a saucepan. Add the bay leaf, fried dhal pieces, the fried onion paste, ginger paste, garlic paste, chilli powder, turmeric and garam masala. Add enough water to cover the dhal pieces. Mix well and simmer for 7-8 minutes.
- Garnish with the coriander leaves. Serve hot.

Varan

(Simple Split Red Gram Dhal)

Serves 4

Ingredients

300g/10oz toor dhal*

2.4 litres/4 pints water

¼ tsp asafoetida

½ tsp turmeric

Salt to taste

Method

- Cook all the ingredients in a saucepan for about 1 hour on a medium heat.
- Serve hot with steamed rice

Sweet Dhal

(Sweet Split Red Gram)

Serves 4-6

Ingredients

300g/10oz toor dhal*

2.5 litres/4 pints water

Salt to taste

¼ tsp turmeric

A large pinch of asafoetida

½ tsp chilli powder

5cm/2in piece of jaggery*

2 tsp refined vegetable oil

¼ tsp cumin seeds

¼ tsp mustard seeds

2 dry red chillies

1 tbsp coriander leaves, finely chopped

Method

- Wash and cook the toor dhal with the water and salt in a saucepan on a low heat for 1 hour.
- Add the turmeric, asafoetida, chilli powder, and jaggery. Cook for 5 minutes. Mix thoroughly. Set aside.
- In a small saucepan, heat the oil. Add the cumin seeds, mustard seeds and the dry red chillies. Let them splutter for 15 seconds.
- Pour this in the dhal and mix well.
- Garnish with the coriander leaves. Serve hot.

Sweet & Sour Dhal

(Sweet and Sour Split Red Gram)

Serves 4-6

Ingredients

300g/10oz toor dhal*

2.4 litres/4 pints water

Salt to taste

¼ tsp turmeric

¼ tsp asafoetida

1 tsp tamarind paste

1 tsp sugar

2 tsp refined vegetable oil

½ tsp mustard seeds

2 green chillies

8 curry leaves

1 tbsp coriander leaves, finely chopped

Method

- Cook the toor dhal in a saucepan with the water and salt on a medium heat for 1 hour.
- Add the turmeric, asafoetida, tamarind paste and sugar. Cook for 5 minutes. Set aside.
- In a small saucepan, heat the oil. Add the mustard seeds, green chillies and curry leaves. Let them splutter for 15 seconds.
- Pour this seasoning in the dhal.
- Garnish with the coriander leaves.
- Serve hot with steamed rice or chapattis

Mung-ni-Dhal

(Split Green Gram)

Serves 4

Ingredients

300g/10oz mung dhal*

1.9 litres/3½ pints water

Salt to taste

¼ tsp turmeric

½ tsp ginger paste

1 green chilli, finely chopped

¼ tsp sugar

1 tbsp ghee

½ tsp sesame seeds

1 small onion, chopped

1 garlic clove, chopped

Method

- Boil the mung dhal with the water and salt in a saucepan on a medium heat for 30 minutes.
- Add the turmeric, ginger paste, green chilli and sugar. Stir well.
- Add 120ml/4fl oz water if the dhal is dry. Simmer for 2-3 minutes and set aside.
- Heat the ghee in a small saucepan. Add the sesame seeds, onion and garlic. Fry them for 1 minute, stirring continuously.
- Add this to the dhal. Serve hot.

Dhal with Onion & Coconut

(Split Red Gram with Onion and Coconut)

Serves 4-6

Ingredients

300g/10oz toor dhal*

2.8 litres/5 pints water

2 green chillies, chopped

1 small onion, chopped

Salt to taste

¼ tsp turmeric

1½ tsp vegetable oil

½ tsp mustard seeds

1 tbsp coriander leaves, finely chopped

50g/1¾oz fresh coconut, grated

Method

- Boil the toor dhal with water, green chillies, onion, salt and turmeric in a saucepan on a medium heat for 1 hour. Set aside.
- Heat the oil in a saucepan. Add the mustard seeds. Let them splutter for 15 seconds.
- Pour this in the dhal and mix well.
- Garnish with the coriander leaves and coconut. Serve hot.

Dahi Kadhi

(Yoghurt-based Curry)

Serves 4

Ingredients

1 tbsp besan*

250g/9oz yoghurt

750ml/1¼ pints water

2 tsp sugar

Salt to taste

½ tsp ginger paste

1 tbsp refined vegetable oil

¼ tsp mustard seeds

¼ tsp cumin seeds

¼ tsp fenugreek seeds

8 curry leaves

10g/¼oz coriander leaves, finely chopped

Method

- Mix the besan with the yoghurt, water, sugar, salt and ginger paste in a large saucepan. Stir well to make sure no lumps form.
- Cook the mixture on a medium heat till it starts to thicken, stirring frequently. Bring to the boil. Set aside.
- Heat the oil in a saucepan. Add the mustard seeds, cumin seeds, fenugreek seeds and curry leaves. Let them splutter for 15 seconds.
- Pour this oil on top of the besan mixture.
- Garnish with the coriander leaves. Serve hot.

Spinach Dhal

(Spinach with Split Green Gram)

Serves 4

Ingredients

300g/10oz mung dhal*

1.9 litres/3½ pints water

Salt to taste

1 large onion, chopped

6 garlic cloves, chopped

¼ tsp turmeric

100g/3½oz spinach, chopped

½ tsp amchoor*

Pinch of garam masala

½ tsp ginger paste

1 tbsp refined vegetable oil

1 tsp cumin seeds

2 tbsp coriander leaves, finely chopped

Method

- Cook the dhal with the water and salt in a saucepan on a medium heat for 30-40 minutes.
- Add the onion and garlic. Cook for 7 minutes.
- Add the turmeric, spinach, amchoor, garam masala and ginger paste. Mix thoroughly.
- Simmer till the dhal is soft and all the spices have been absorbed. Set aside.
- Heat the oil in a saucepan. Add the cumin seeds. Let them splutter for 15 seconds.
- Pour this on top of the dhal.
- Garnish with the coriander leaves. Serve hot

Tawker Dhal

(Sour Split Red Lentil with Unripe Mango)

Serves 4

Ingredients

300g/10oz toor dhal*

2.4 litres/4 pints water

1 unripe mango, stoned and quartered

½ tsp turmeric

4 green chillies

Salt to taste

2 tsp mustard oil

½ tsp mustard seeds

1 tbsp coriander leaves, finely chopped

Method
- Boil the dhal with the water, mango pieces, turmeric, green chillies and salt for an hour. Set aside.
- Heat the oil in a saucepan and add the mustard seeds. Let them splutter for 15 seconds.
- Add this to the dhal. Simmer till thick.
- Garnish with the coriander leaves.
  Serve hot with steamed rice

Basic Dhal

(Split Red Gram with Tomato)

Serves 4

Ingredients

300g/10oz toor dhal*

1.2 litres/2 pints water

Salt to taste

¼ tsp turmeric

½ tbsp refined vegetable oil

¼ tsp cumin seeds

2 green chillies, slit lengthways

1 medium-sized tomato, finely chopped

1 tbsp coriander leaves, finely chopped

Method

- Cook the toor dhal with the water and salt in a saucepan for 1 hour on a medium heat.
- Add the turmeric and mix well.
- If the dhal is too thick, add 120ml/4fl oz water to it. Mix well and set aside.
- Heat the oil in a saucepan. Add the cumin seeds and let them splutter for 15 seconds. Add the green chillies and tomato. Fry for 2 minutes.
- Add this to the dhal. Mix and simmer for 3 minutes.
- Garnish with the coriander leaves. Serve hot with steamed rice

Maa-ki-Dhal

(Rich Black Gram)

Serves 4

Ingredients

240g kaali dhal*

125g/4½oz kidney beans

2.8 litres/5 pints water

Salt to taste

3.5cm/1½in root ginger, julienned

1 tsp chilli powder

3 tomatoes, puréed

1 tbsp butter

2 tsp refined vegetable oil

1 tsp cumin seeds

2 tbsp single cream

Method
- Soak the dhal and the kidney beans together overnight.
- Cook with the water, salt and ginger in a saucepan for 40 minutes on a medium heat.
- Add the chilli powder, tomato purée and butter. Simmer for 8-10 minutes. Set aside.
- Heat the oil in a saucepan. Add the cumin seeds. Let them splutter for 15 seconds.
- Add this to the dhal. Mix well.
- Add the cream. Serve hot with steamed rice

Dhansak

(Spicy Parsi Split Red Gram)

Serves 4

Ingredients

3 tbsp refined vegetable oil

1 large onion, finely chopped

2 large tomatoes, chopped

½ tsp turmeric

½ tsp chilli powder

1 tbsp dhansak masala*

1 tbsp malt vinegar

Salt to taste

For the dhal mixture:

150g/5½oz toor dhal*

75g/2½oz mung dhal*

75g/2½oz masoor dhal*

1 small aubergine, quartered

7.5cm/3in piece of pumpkin, quartered

1 tbsp fresh fenugreek leaves

1.4 litres/2½ pints water

Salt to taste

Method

- Cook the ingredients for the dhal mixture together in a saucepan on a medium heat for 45 minutes. Set aside.
- Heat the oil in a saucepan. Fry the onions and tomatoes on a medium heat for 2-3 minutes.
- Add the dhal mixture and all the remaining ingredients. Mix well and cook on a medium heat for 5-7 minutes. Serve hot.

Masoor Dhal

Serves 4

Ingredients

300g/10oz masoor dhal*

Salt to taste

Pinch of turmeric

1.2 litres/2 pints water

2 tbsp refined vegetable oil

6 garlic cloves, crushed

1 tsp lemon juice

Method

- Cook the dhal, salt, turmeric and water in a saucepan on a medium heat for 45 minutes. Set aside.
- Heat the oil in a frying pan and fry the garlic till brown. Add to the dhal and sprinkle with the lemon juice. Mix well. Serve hot.

Panchemel Dhal

(Five Lentil Mix)

Serves 4

Ingredients

75g/2½oz mung dhal*

1 tbsp chana dhal*

1 tbsp masoor dhal*

1 tbsp toor dhal*

1 tbsp urad dhal*

750ml/1¼ pints water

½ tsp turmeric

Salt to taste

1 tbsp ghee

1 tsp cumin seeds

Pinch of asafoetida

½ tsp garam masala

1 tsp ginger paste

Method

- Cook the dhals with the water, turmeric and salt in a saucepan for 1 hour on a medium heat. Stir well. Set aside.
- Heat the ghee in a saucepan. Fry the remaining ingredients for 1 minute.
- Add this to the dhal, mix well and simmer for 3-4 minutes. Serve hot.

Cholar Dhal

(Split Bengal Gram)

Serves 4

Ingredients

600g/1lb 5oz chana dhal*

2.4 litres/5 pints water

Salt to taste

3 tbsp ghee

½ tsp cumin seeds

½ tsp turmeric

2 tsp sugar

3 cloves

2 bay leaves

2.5cm/1in cinnamon

2 green cardamom pods

15g/½oz coconut, chopped and fried

Method
- Cook the dhal with the water and salt in a saucepan on a medium heat for 1 hour. Set aside.
- Heat 2 tbsp ghee in a saucepan. Add all the ingredients, except the coconut. Let them splutter for 20 seconds. Add the cooked dhal and cook, stirring well for 5 minutes. Add the coconut and 1 tbsp ghee. Serve hot.

Dilpasand Dhal

(Special Lentils)

Serves 4

Ingredients

60g/2oz urad beans*

2 tbsp kidney beans

2 tbsp chickpeas

2 litres/3½ pints water

¼ tsp turmeric

2 tbsp ghee

2 tomatoes, blanched and puréed

2 tsp ground cumin, dry roasted

125g/4½oz yoghurt, whisked

120ml/4fl oz single cream

Salt to taste

Method

- Mix both the beans, chickpeas and water. Soak in a saucepan for 4 hours. Add the turmeric and cook for 45 minutes on a medium heat. Set aside.
- Heat the ghee in a saucepan. Add all the remaining ingredients and cook on a medium heat till the ghee separates.
- Add the beans and chickpeas mixture. Simmer till dry. Serve hot.

Dhal Masoor

(Split Red Lentils)

Serves 4

Ingredients

1 tbsp ghee

1 tsp cumin seeds

1 small onion, finely chopped

2.5cm/1in root ginger, finely chopped

6 garlic cloves, finely chopped

4 green chillies, slit lengthways

1 tomato, peeled and puréed

½ tsp turmeric

300g/10oz masoor dhal*

1.5 litres/2¾ pints water

Salt to taste

2 tbsp coriander leaves

Method

- Heat the ghee in a saucepan. Add the cumin seeds, onion, ginger, garlic, chillies, tomato and turmeric. Fry for 5 minutes, stirring frequently.
- Add the dhal, water and salt. Simmer for 45 minutes. Garnish with the coriander leaves. Serve hot with steamed rice

Dhal with Aubergine

(Lentils with Aubergine)

Serves 4

Ingredients

300g/10oz toor dhal*

1.5 litre/2¾ pints water

Salt to taste

1 tbsp refined vegetable oil

50g/1¾oz aubergines, diced

2.5cm/1in cinnamon

2 green cardamom pods

2 cloves

1 large onion, finely chopped

2 large tomatoes, finely chopped

½ tsp ginger paste

½ tsp garlic paste

1 tsp ground coriander

½ tsp turmeric

10g/¼oz coriander leaves, to garnish

Method

- Boil the dhal with the water and salt in a saucepan for 45 minutes on a medium heat. Set aside.
- Heat the oil in a saucepan. Add all the remaining ingredients, except the coriander leaves. Fry for 2-3 minutes, stirring constantly.
- Add the mixture to the dhal. Simmer for 5 minutes. Garnish and serve.

Yellow Dhal Tadka

Serves 4

Ingredients

300g/10oz mung dhal*

1 litre/1¾ pints water

¼ tsp turmeric

Salt to taste

3 tsp ghee

½ tsp mustard seeds

½ tsp cumin seeds

½ tsp fenugreek seeds

2.5cm/1in root ginger, finely chopped

4 garlic cloves, finely chopped

3 green chillies, slit lengthways

8 curry leaves

Method

- Cook the dhal with the water, turmeric and salt in a saucepan for 45 minutes on a medium heat. Set aside.
- Heat the ghee in a saucepan. Add all the remaining ingredients. Fry them for 1 minute and pour on top of the dhal. Mix well and serve hot.

Rasam

(Spicy Tamarind-based Soup)

Serves 4

Ingredients

2 tbsp tamarind paste

750ml/1¼ pints water

8-10 curry leaves

2 tbsp chopped coriander leaves

Pinch of asafoetida

Salt to taste

2 tsp ghee

½ tsp mustard seeds

For the spice mixture:

2 tsp coriander seeds

2 tbsp toor dhal*

1 tsp cumin seeds

4-5 peppercorns

1 dried red chilli

Method

- Dry roast and grind the spice mixture ingredients together.
- Mix the spice mixture with all the ingredients, except the ghee and the mustard seeds. Cook for 7 minutes on a medium heat in a saucepan.
- Heat the ghee in another saucepan. Add the mustard seeds and let them splutter for 15 seconds. Pour this directly in the rasam. Serve hot.

Simple Mung Dhal

Serves 4

Ingredients

300g/10oz mung dhal*

1 litre/1¾ pints water

Pinch of turmeric

Salt to taste

2 tbsp refined vegetable oil

1 large onion, finely chopped

3 green chillies, finely chopped

2.5cm/1in root ginger, finely chopped

5 curry leaves

2 tomatoes, finely chopped

Method

- Cook the dhal with the water, turmeric and salt in a saucepan for 30 minutes on a medium heat. Set aside.
- Heat the oil in a saucepan. Add all the remaining ingredients. Fry for 3-4 minutes. Add this to the dhal. Simmer till thick. Serve hot.

Whole Green Mung

Serves 4

Ingredients

250g/9oz mung beans, soaked overnight

1 litre/1¾ pints water

½ tbsp refined vegetable oil

½ tsp cumin seeds

6 curry leaves

1 large onion, finely chopped

½ tsp garlic paste

½ tsp ginger paste

3 green chillies, finely chopped

1 tomato, finely chopped

¼ tsp turmeric

Salt to taste

120ml/4fl oz milk

Method
- Cook the beans with the water in a saucepan for 45 minutes on a medium heat. Set aside.
- Heat the oil in a saucepan. Add the cumin seeds and curry leaves.
- After 15 seconds, add the cooked beans and all the remaining ingredients. Mix well and simmer for 7-8 minutes. Serve hot.

Dahi Kadhi with Pakoras

(Yoghurt-based Curry with Fried Dumplings)

Serves 4

Ingredients
For the pakora:

125g/4½oz besan*

¼ tsp cumin seeds

2 tsp chopped onions

1 chopped green chilli

½ tsp grated ginger

Pinch of turmeric

2 green chillies, finely chopped

½ tsp ajowan seeds

Salt to taste

Oil for deep frying

For the kadhi:
Dahi Kadhi

Method

- In a bowl, mix all the pakora ingredients, except the oil, with enough water to form a thick batter. Fry spoonfuls in hot oil till golden brown.
- Cook the kadhi and add the pakoras to it. Simmer for 3-4 minutes.
- Serve hot with steamed rice

Sweet Unripe Mango Dhal

(Split Red Gram with Unripe Mango)

Serves 4

Ingredients

300g/10oz toor dhal*

2 green chillies, slit lengthways

2 tsp jaggery*, grated

1 small onion, sliced

Salt to taste

¼ tsp turmeric

1.5 litres/2¾ pints water

1 unripe mango, peeled and chopped

1½ tsp refined vegetable oil

½ tsp mustard seeds

1 tbsp coriander leaves, for garnish

Method

- Mix all the ingredients, except the oil, mustard seeds and coriander leaves, in a saucepan. Cook for 30 minutes on a medium heat. Set aside.
- Heat the oil in a saucepan. Add the mustard seeds. Let them splutter for 15 seconds. Pour this on top of the dhal. Garnish and serve hot.

Malai Dhal

(Split Black Gram with Cream)

Serves 4

Ingredients

300g/10oz urad dhal*, soaked for 4 hours

1 litre/1¾ pints water

500ml/16fl oz milk, boiled

1 tsp turmeric

Salt to taste

½ tsp amchoor*

2 tbsp single cream

1 tbsp ghee

1 tsp cumin seeds

2.5cm/1in root ginger, finely chopped

1 small tomato, finely chopped

1 small onion, finely chopped

Method
- Cook the dhal with the water on a medium heat for 45 minutes.
- Add the milk, turmeric, salt, amchoor and cream. Mix well and cook for 3-4 minutes. Set aside.
- Heat the ghee in a saucepan. Add the cumin seeds, ginger, tomato and onion. Fry for 3 minutes. Add this to the dhal. Mix well and serve hot.

Sambhar

(Mixed Lentils and Vegetables cooked with special spices)

Serves 4

Ingredients

300g/10oz toor dhal*

1.5 litres/2¾ pints water

Salt to taste

1 tbsp refined vegetable oil

1 large onion, thinly sliced

2 tsp tamarind paste

¼ tsp turmeric

1 green chilli, roughly chopped

1½ tsp sambhar powder*

2 tbsp coriander leaves, finely chopped

For the seasoning:

1 green chilli, slit lengthways

1 tsp mustard seeds

½ tsp urad dhal*

8 curry leaves

¼ tsp asafoetida

Method

- Mix all the ingredients of the seasoning together. Set aside.
- Cook the toor dhal with the water and salt in a saucepan on a medium heat for 40 minutes. Mash well. Set aside.
- Heat the oil in a saucepan. Add the seasoning ingredients. Let them splutter for 20 seconds.
- Add the cooked dhal and all the remaining ingredients, except the coriander leaves. Cook on a low heat for 8-10 minutes.
- Garnish with the coriander leaves. Serve hot.

Three Dhals

(Mixed Lentils)

Serves 4

Ingredients

150g/5½oz toor dhal*

75g/2½oz masoor dhal*

75g/2½oz mung dhal*

1 litre/1¾ pints water

1 large tomato, finely chopped

1 small onion, finely chopped

4 garlic cloves, finely chopped

6 curry leaves

Salt to taste

¼ tsp turmeric

2 tbsp refined vegetable oil

½ tsp cumin seeds

Method
- Soak the dhals in the water for 30 minutes. Cook with the remaining ingredients, except the oil and cumin, for 45 minutes on a medium heat.
- Heat the oil in a saucepan. Add the cumin seeds. Let them splutter for 15 seconds. Pour this on top of the dhal. Mix well. Serve hot.

Methi-Drumstick Sambhar

(Fenugreek and Drumsticks with Split Red Gram)

Serves 4

Ingredients

300g/10oz toor dhal*

1 litre/1¾ pints water

Pinch of turmeric

Salt to taste

2 Indian drumsticks*, chopped

1 tsp refined vegetable oil

¼ tsp mustard seeds

1 red chilli, halved

¼ tsp asafoetida

10g/¼oz fresh fenugreek leaves, chopped

1¼ tsp sambhar powder*

1¼ tsp tamarind paste

Method

- Mix the dhal, water, turmeric, salt and drumsticks in a saucepan. Cook for 45 minutes on a medium heat. Set aside.
- Heat the oil in a pan. Add all the remaining ingredients and stir-fry for 2-3 minutes. Add this to the dhal and simmer for 7-8 minutes. Serve hot.

Dhal Shorba

(Lentil Soup)

Serves 4

Ingredients

300g/10oz toor dhal*

Salt to taste

1 litre/1¾ pints water

1 tbsp refined vegetable oil

2 large onions, sliced

4 garlic cloves, crushed

50g/1¾oz spinach leaves, finely chopped

3 tomatoes, finely chopped

1 tsp lemon juice

1 tsp garam masala

Method

- Cook the dhal, salt and water in a saucepan on a medium heat for 45 minutes. Set aside.
- Heat the oil. Fry the onions on a medium heat till brown. Add all the remaining ingredients and cook for 5 minutes, stirring frequently.
- Add this to the dhal mixture. Serve hot.

Yummy Mung

(Whole Mung)

Serves 4

Ingredients

250g/9oz mung beans

2.5 litres/4 pints water

Salt to taste

2 medium-sized onions, chopped

3 green chillies, chopped

¼ tsp turmeric

1 tsp chilli powder

1 tsp lemon juice

1 tbsp refined vegetable oil

½ tsp cumin seeds

6 garlic cloves, crushed

Method

- Soak the mung beans in the water for 3-4 hours. Cook in a saucepan with the salt, onions, green chillies, turmeric and chilli powder on a medium heat for 1 hour.
- Add the lemon juice. Simmer for 10 minutes. Set aside.
- Heat the oil in a saucepan. Add the cumin seeds and garlic. Fry for 1 minute on a medium heat. Pour this in the mung mixture. Serve hot.

Masala Toor Dhal

(Spicy Split Red Gram)

Serves 4

Ingredients

300g/10oz toor dhal*

1.5 litres/2¾ pints water

Salt to taste

½ tsp turmeric

1 tbsp refined vegetable oil

½ tsp mustard seeds

8 curry leaves

¼ tsp asafoetida

½ tsp ginger paste

½ tsp garlic paste

1 green chilli, finely chopped

1 onion, finely chopped

1 tomato, finely chopped

2 tsp lemon juice

2 tbsp coriander leaves, to garnish

Method

- Cook the dhal with the water, salt and turmeric in a saucepan for 45 minutes on a medium heat. Set aside.
- Heat the oil in a saucepan. Add all the ingredients, except the lemon juice and coriander leaves. Fry for 3-4 minutes on a medium heat. Pour this on top of the dhal.
- Add the lemon juice and coriander leaves. Mix well. Serve hot.

Dry Yellow Mung Dhal

(Dry Yellow Gram)

Serves 4

Ingredients

300g/10oz mung dhal*, soaked for 1 hour

250ml/8fl oz water

¼ tsp turmeric

Salt to taste

1 tbsp ghee

1 tsp amchoor*

1 tbsp coriander leaves, chopped

1 small onion, finely chopped

Method

- Cook the dhal with the water, turmeric and salt in a saucepan for 45 minutes on a medium heat.
- Heat the ghee and pour it on top of the dhal. Sprinkle the amchoor, coriander leaves and the onion on top. Serve hot.

Whole Urad

(Whole Black Gram)

Serves 4

Ingredients

300g/10oz urad beans*, washed

Salt to taste

1.25 litres/2½ pints water

¼ tsp turmeric

½ tsp chilli powder

½ tsp dried ginger powder

¾ tsp garam masala

1 tbsp ghee

½ tsp cumin seeds

1 large onion, finely chopped

2 tbsp coriander leaves, finely chopped

Method

- Cook the urad beans with the salt and water in a saucepan for 45 minutes on a medium heat.
- Add the turmeric, chilli powder, ginger powder and garam masala. Mix well and simmer for 5 minutes. Set aside.
- Heat the ghee in a saucepan. Add the cumin seeds and let them splutter for 15 seconds. Add the onion and fry it on a medium heat till brown.
- Add the onion mixture to the dhal and mix well. Simmer for 10 minutes.
- Garnish with the coriander leaves. Serve hot.

Dhal Fry

(Split Red Gram with Fried Spices)

Serves 4

Ingredients

300g/10oz toor dhal*

1.5 litres/2¾ pints water

½ tsp turmeric

Salt to taste

2 tbsp ghee

½ tsp mustard seeds

½ tsp cumin seeds

½ tsp fenugreek seeds

2.5cm/1in root ginger, finely chopped

2-3 garlic cloves, finely chopped

2 green chillies, finely chopped

1 small onion, finely chopped

1 tomato, finely chopped

Method

- Cook the dhal with the water, turmeric and salt in a saucepan for 45 minutes over a medium heat. Stir well. Set aside.
- Heat the ghee in a saucepan. Add the mustard seeds, cumin seeds and fenugreek seeds. Let them splutter for 15 seconds.
- Add the ginger, garlic, green chillies, onion and tomato. Fry on a medium heat for 3-4 minutes, stirring frequently. Add this to the dhal. Serve hot.

Kale Moti ki Biryani

(Whole Black Gram Biryani)

Serves 4

Ingredients

500g/1lb 2oz basmati rice, soaked for 30 minutes and drained

500ml/16fl oz milk

1 tsp garam masala

500ml/16fl oz water

Salt to taste

75g/2½oz ghee

2 tsp ginger paste

2 tsp garlic paste

3 green chillies, slit lengthways

6 large potatoes, peeled and quartered

2 tomatoes, finely chopped

½ tsp chilli powder

⅓ tsp turmeric

200g/7oz yoghurt

300g/10oz urad beans*, cooked

1 tsp saffron, soaked in 60ml/2fl oz milk

25g/scant 1oz coriander leaves, finely chopped

10g/¼oz mint leaves, finely chopped

2 large onions, sliced and deep fried

3 green cardamom pods

5 cloves

2.5cm/1in cinnamon

1 bay leaf

Method

- Cook the rice with the milk, garam masala, water and salt in a saucepan on a medium heat for 7-8 minutes. Set aside.
- Heat the ghee in an ovenproof dish. Add the ginger paste and garlic paste. Stir-fry on a medium heat for a minute.
- Add the green chillies and potatoes. Fry the mixture for 3-4 minutes.
- Add the tomatoes, chilli powder and turmeric. Mix well. Fry for 2-3 minutes, stirring frequently.
- Add the yoghurt. Stir thoroughly for 2-3 minutes.
- Add the urad beans. Cook on a low heat for 7-10 minutes.
- Sprinkle the coriander leaves, mint leaves, onions, cardamom, cloves, cinnamon and bay leaf over the beans.

- Spread the cooked rice evenly over the beans mixture. Pour the saffron milk over the rice.
- Seal with foil and cover with a lid.
- Bake the biryani in an oven at 200°C (400°F, Gas Mark 6) for 15-20 minutes. Serve hot.

Mince & Masoor Pulao

(Mince and Whole Red Lentil with Pilau Rice)

Serves 4

Ingredients

6 tbsp refined vegetable oil

2 cloves

2 green cardamom pods

6 black peppercorns

2 bay leaves

2.5cm/1in cinnamon

1 tsp ginger paste

1 tsp garlic paste

1 large onion, finely chopped

2 green chillies, finely chopped

1 tsp chilli powder

½ tsp turmeric

2 tsp ground coriander

1 tsp ground cumin

500g/1lb 2oz lamb mince

150g/5½oz whole masoor*, soaked for 30 minutes and drained

250g/9oz long-grained rice, soaked for 30 minutes and drained

750ml/1¼ pints hot water

Salt to taste

10g/¼oz coriander leaves, finely chopped

Method

- Heat the oil in a saucepan. Add the cloves, cardamom, peppercorns, bay leaves, cinnamon, ginger paste and garlic paste. Fry this mixture on a medium heat for 2-3 minutes.
- Add the onion. Stir-fry till it turns translucent.
- Add the green chillies. Fry for a minute.
- Add the chilli powder, turmeric, ground coriander and cumin. Stir for 2 minutes.
- Add the mince, masoor and rice. Fry well on a medium heat for 5 minutes, stirring lightly at regular intervals.
- Add the hot water and the salt.
- Cover with a lid and simmer for 15 minutes.
- Garnish the pulao with the coriander leaves. Serve hot.

Chicken Biryani

Serves 4

Ingredients

1kg/2¼lb skinned chicken with the bones, cut into 8 pieces

6 tbsp refined vegetable oil

10 cashew nuts

10 raisins

500g/1lb 2oz basmati rice, soaked for 30 minutes and drained

3 cloves

2 bay leaves

5cm/2in cinnamon

4 black peppercorns

Salt to taste

4 large onions, finely sliced

250ml/8fl oz water

2½ tbsp ghee

A large pinch of saffron, dissolved in 1 tbsp milk

For the marinade:

1½ tsp garlic paste

1½ tsp ginger paste

3 green chillies, finely chopped

1 tsp garam masala

1 tsp ground black pepper

1 tbsp ground coriander

2 tsp ground cumin

125g/4½oz yoghurt

Method

- Mix all the marinade ingredients together. Marinate the chicken with this mixture for 3-4 hours.
- Heat 1 tbsp oil in a small saucepan. Add the cashew nuts and raisins. Fry on a medium heat till brown. Drain and set aside.
- Parboil the drained rice with the cloves, bay leaves, cinnamon, peppercorns and salt. Set aside.
- Heat 3 tbsp oil in a saucepan. Add the chicken pieces and fry on a medium heat for 20 minutes, turning occasionally. Set aside.
- Heat the remaining oil in another saucepan. Add the onions and fry them on a medium heat till brown.
- Add the fried chicken pieces. Cook them for 5 more minutes on a medium heat.
- Add the water and simmer till the chicken is cooked. Set aside.
- Pour 2 tbsp ghee in an ovenproof dish. Add the chicken mixture. Arrange the rice in a layer over the chicken.
- Pour the saffron milk on top and add the remaining ghee.
- Seal with foil and cover tightly with a lid.

- Bake in an oven at 200°C (400°F, Gas Mark 6) for 8-10 minutes.
- Garnish with the fried cashew nuts and raisins. Serve hot.

Prawn Biryani

Serves 6

Ingredients

600g/1lb 5oz big prawns, cleaned and de-veined

Salt to taste

1 tsp turmeric

250ml/8fl oz refined vegetable oil

4 large onions, sliced

4 tomatoes, finely chopped

2-3 potatoes, peeled and diced

50g/1¾oz coriander leaves, finely chopped

25g/scant 1oz mint leaves, finely chopped

200g/7oz yoghurt

2 green chillies, chopped

450g/1lb steamed basmati rice (see here)

For the spice mixture:

4 cloves

2.5cm/1in cinnamon

3 green cardamom pods

4 black peppercorns

2-3 green chillies

¼ fresh coconut, grated

4 red chillies

12 garlic cloves

1 tsp cumin

1 tsp coriander

Method

- Coarsely grind together all the spice mixture ingredients. Set aside.
- Mix the prawns with the salt and turmeric. Set aside.
- Heat 2 tbsp of the oil in a saucepan. Add the onions and fry them on a medium heat till they turn brown. Set aside.
- Heat the remaining oil in a saucepan. Add half of the fried onions along with the ground spice mixture. Mix well and fry on a medium heat for a minute.
- Add the tomatoes, potatoes, salt and the prawns. Cook the mixture for 5 minutes.
- Add the coriander, mint leaves, yoghurt and green chillies. Mix well. Simmer for 10 minutes, stirring lightly at frequent intervals. Set aside.
- In a large saucepan, arrange the rice and prawn mixture in alternate layers. End with a layer of rice.
- Sprinkle the remaining onions over it, cover with a lid and simmer for 30 minutes. Serve hot.

Egg Potato Biryani

Serves 4-5

Ingredients

5 tbsp refined vegetable oil

3 cloves

2.5cm/1in cinnamon

3 green cardamom pods

2 bay leaves

6 peppercorns

3 large onions, finely sliced

3 large tomatoes, finely chopped

Salt to taste

¼ tsp turmeric

200g/7oz yoghurt

3 large potatoes, peeled, quartered and deep fried

6 eggs, boiled and halved lengthways

300g/10oz steamed basmati rice

2 tbsp ghee

1 tbsp cumin seeds

Dash of yellow food colour

For the paste:

1 tbsp white sesame seeds

4-5 red chillies

8 garlic cloves

5cm/2in root ginger

2-3 green chillies

50g/1¾oz coriander leaves

1 tbsp coriander seeds

Method

- Grind together all the paste ingredients with enough water to form a thick paste. Set aside.
- Heat the oil in a saucepan. Add all the cloves, cinnamon, cardamom, bay leaves and peppercorns. Let them splutter for 30 seconds.
- Add the onions. Fry them on a medium heat till they turn translucent.
- Add the paste with the tomatoes, salt and turmeric. Fry for 2-3 minutes, stirring ocasionally.
- Add the yoghurt. Cook the mixture on a medium heat, stirring frequently.
- Add the potatoes. Toss them well to coat them with the sauce.
- Gently add the egg pieces, yolk side up.
- Spread the rice over the egg pieces. Set this arrangement aside.
- Heat the ghee in a small saucepan. Add the cumin seeds. Let them splutter for 15 seconds.

- Pour this mixture directly on top of the rice arrangement.
- Sprinkle the food colour over it and cover the pan with a lid.
- Simmer for 30 minutes. Serve hot.

Mince Pulao

(Minced Lamb with Pilau Rice)

Serves 4

Ingredients

5 tbsp refined vegetable oil

2 cloves

2 green cardamom pods

6 black peppercorns

2 bay leaves

2.5cm/1in cinnamon

1 large onion, finely chopped

1 tsp ginger paste

1 tsp garlic paste

2 green chillies, finely chopped

2 tsp ground coriander

1 tsp chilli powder

½ tsp turmeric

1 tsp ground cumin

500g/1lb 2oz lamb mince

350g/12oz long-grained rice, soaked for 30 minutes in water and drained

750 ml/1¼fl oz hot water

Salt to taste

10g/¼oz coriander leaves, finely chopped

Method

- Heat the oil in a saucepan. Add the cloves, cardamom, peppercorns, bay leaves and cinnamon. Let them splutter for 15 seconds.
- Add the onion. Fry on a medium heat till translucent.
- Add the ginger paste, garlic paste, green chillies, ground coriander, chilli powder, turmeric and ground cumin.
- Fry for 2 minutes. Add the mince and rice. Stir-fry this mixture for 5 minutes.
- Add the hot water and the salt.
- Cover with a lid and simmer for 15 minutes.
- Garnish the pulao with the coriander leaves. Serve hot.

Chana Pulao

(Chickpeas with Pilau Rice)

Serves 4

Ingredients

2 tbsp refined vegetable oil

1 tsp cumin seeds

1 large onion, finely chopped

1 tsp ginger paste

1 tsp garlic paste

2 green chillies, finely chopped

300g/10oz canned chickpeas

300g/10oz long-grained rice, soaked for 30 minutes and drained

Salt to taste

250ml/8fl oz water

Method

- Heat the oil in a saucepan. Add the cumin seeds. Let them splutter for 15 seconds.
- Add the onion, ginger paste, garlic paste and green chillies. Fry this mixture on a medium heat for 2-3 minutes.

- Add the chickpeas and rice. Stir-fry for 4-5 minutes.
- Add the salt and the water. Cook the pulao on a medium heat for a minute.
- Cover with a lid and simmer for 10-12 minutes.
- Serve hot.

Simple Khichdi

(Rice and Lentil Melange)

Serves 4

Ingredients

1 tbsp ghee

1 tsp cumin seeds

2 green chillies, slit lengthways

250g/9oz long-grained rice

150g/5½oz mung dhal*

1 litre/1¾ pints hot water

Salt to taste

Method

- Heat the ghee in a saucepan. Add the cumin seeds and green chillies. Let them splutter for 15 seconds.
- Add the rice and mung dhal. Stir-fry for 5 minutes.
- Add the hot water and salt. Mix well. Cover with a lid. Simmer the khichdi for 15 minutes – it should have a porridge-like consistency.
- Serve hot.

Masala Rice

(Spicy Rice)

Serves 4

Ingredients

6 tbsp refined vegetable oil

½ tsp mustard seeds

10 curry leaves

2 green chillies, slit lengthways

¼ tsp turmeric

2 large onions, finely sliced

½ tsp chilli powder

2 tsp lemon juice

Salt to taste

300g/10oz steamed long-grained rice

1 tbsp coriander leaves, chopped

Method

- Heat the oil in a saucepan. Add the mustard seeds, curry leaves and green chillies. Let them splutter for 15 seconds. Add the turmeric and the onions. Fry the mixture on a medium heat till the onions are brown.
- Add the remaining ingredients, except the coriander. Stir gently over a low heat for 5 minutes. Garnish with the coriander leaves. Serve hot.

Onion Rice

Serves 4

Ingredients

5 tbsp refined vegetable oil

½ tsp mustard seeds

½ tsp cumin

4 medium-sized onions, finely sliced

3 green chillies, finely chopped

5 garlic cloves, finely chopped

300g/10oz steamed basmati rice

Salt to taste

60ml/2fl oz water

10g/¼oz coriander leaves, chopped

Method

- Heat the oil in a saucepan. Add the mustard seeds and cumin. Let them splutter for 15 seconds.
- Add the onions, green chillies and garlic. Fry this mixture on a medium heat till the onions are translucent.

- Add the rice, salt and water. Cook on a medium heat for 5-7 minutes.
- Garnish the onion rice with the coriander leaves. Serve hot.

Steamed Rice

Serves 4

Ingredients

375g/13oz long-grained or basmati rice

750ml/1¼ pints water

Method

- Wash the rice well.
- Heat the water in a saucepan. Add the rice and cook on a high heat for 8-10 minutes.
- Press a grain of rice lightly between your thumb and your forefinger to check if it is cooked.
- Remove from the heat and drain in a colander. Serve hot.

Stuffed Aubergines

Serves 4

Ingredients

10 small aubergines

1 large onion, finely chopped

3 tbsp fresh coconut, grated

1 tsp ground cumin

1 tsp chilli powder

50g/1¾oz coriander leaves, chopped

Juice of 1 lemon

Salt to taste

3 tbsp refined vegetable oil

Method

- Make a cross with a knife at one end of each aubergine and slit, not severing the other end. Set aside.

- Mix the remaining ingredients, except the oil. Stuff this mixture in the slit aubergines.

- Heat the oil in a frying pan. Add the aubergines and fry them on a medium heat for 3-4 minutes. Cover and cook for 10 minutes, carefully turning the aubergines occasionally. Serve hot.

Sarson ka Saag

(Mustard Greens in Sauce)

Serves 4

Ingredients

3 tbsp refined vegetable oil

100g/3½oz mustard leaves, chopped

200g/7oz spinach, finely chopped

3 green chillies, slit lengthways

1cm/½in root ginger, julienned

2 garlic cloves, crushed

Salt to taste

250ml/8fl oz water

2 tbsp ghee

Blob of butter

Method

- Heat the oil in a saucepan. Add the mustard leaves, spinach and green chillies. Fry them on a medium heat for a minute.

- Add the ginger, garlic, salt and water. Mix well. Simmer for 10 minutes.

- Purée the mixture in a blender until smooth.

- Transfer to a saucepan and cook on a medium heat for 15 minutes.

- Garnish with the butter. Serve hot.

Shahi Paneer

(Paneer in Rich Sauce)

Serves 4

Ingredients

4 tbsp refined vegetable oil

500g/1lb 2oz paneer*, chopped

2 large onions, ground to a paste

1 tsp ginger paste

1 tsp garlic paste

1 tsp chilli powder

300g/10oz tomato purée

200g/7oz yoghurt, whisked

250ml/8fl oz single cream

Salt to taste

Method

- Heat 1 tbsp oil in a saucepan. Add the paneer pieces. Fry them on a medium heat till they turn golden brown. Drain and set aside.

- Add the remaining oil in the same pan. Add the onions, ginger paste and garlic paste. Fry for a minute. Add the paneer and the remaining ingredients. Cook for 5 minutes, stirring occasionally. Serve hot.

Tandoori Potato

Serves 4

Ingredients

16 large potatoes, peeled

Refined vegetable oil to deep fry

3 tbsp finely chopped tomatoes

1 tbsp coriander leaves, chopped

1 tsp garam masala

100g/3½oz Cheddar cheese, grated

Salt to taste

Juice of 2 lemons

Method

- Scoop out the potatoes. Reserve the flesh and the hollowed parts.

- Heat the oil in a frying pan. Add the hollowed potatoes. Fry them on a medium heat till they turn golden brown. Set aside.

- To the same oil, add the scooped potatoes and all the remaining ingredients, except the lemon juice. Sauté on a low heat for 5 minutes.

- Stuff this mixture inside the hollow potatoes.

- Bake the stuffed potatoes in an oven at 200°C (400°F, Gas Mark 6) for 5 minutes.

- Sprinkle the lemon juice on top of the potatoes. Serve hot.

Corn Curry

Serves 4

Ingredients

1 large potato, boiled and mashed

500g/1lb 2oz tomato purée

3 tbsp refined vegetable oil

8 curry leaves

2 tbsp besan*

1 tsp ginger paste

½ tsp turmeric

Salt to taste

1 tsp garam masala

1 tsp chilli powder

3 tsp sugar

250ml/8fl oz water

4 corn on the cobs, chopped into 3 pieces each and boiled

Method

- Mix the potato mash thoroughly with the tomato purée. Set aside.

- Heat the oil in a saucepan. Add the curry leaves. Let them crackle for 10 seconds. Add the besan and ginger paste. Fry on a low heat till brown.

- Add the potato-tomato mixture and all the remaining ingredients except the corn. Simmer for 3-4 minutes.

- Add the corn pieces. Mix well. Simmer for 8-10 minutes. Serve hot.

Masala Green Pepper

Serves 4

Ingredients

1½ tbsp refined vegetable oil

1 tsp garam masala

¼ tsp turmeric

½ tsp ginger paste

½ tsp garlic paste

1 large onion, finely chopped

1 tomato, finely chopped

4 large green peppers, julienned

125g/4½oz yoghurt

Salt to taste

Method

- Heat the oil in a saucepan. Add the garam masala, turmeric, ginger paste and garlic paste. Fry this mixture on a medium heat for 2 minutes.

- Add the onion. Fry till it is translucent.

- Add the tomato and green peppers. Fry for 2-3 minutes. Add the yoghurt and salt. Mix well. Cook for 6-7 minutes. Serve hot.

No-oil Bottle Gourd

Serves 4

Ingredients

500g/1lb 2oz bottle gourd*, skinned and chopped

2 tomatoes, finely chopped

1 large onion, finely chopped

1 tsp ginger paste

1 tsp garlic paste

2 green chillies, finely chopped

½ tsp ground coriander

½ tsp ground cumin

25g/scant 1oz coriander leaves, finely chopped

120ml/4fl oz water

Salt to taste

Method

- Mix all the ingredients together. Cook in a saucepan on a low heat for 20 minutes. Serve hot.

Okra with Yoghurt

Serves 4

Ingredients

3 tbsp refined vegetable oil

½ tsp cumin seeds

500g/1lb 2oz okra, chopped

½ tsp chilli powder

¼ tsp turmeric

2 green chillies, slit lengthways

1 tsp ginger, julienned

200g/7oz yoghurt

1 tsp besan*, dissolved in 1 tbsp water

Salt to taste

1 tbsp coriander leaves, finely chopped

Method

- Heat the oil in a saucepan. Add the cumin seeds. Let them splutter for 15 seconds.

- Add the okra, chilli powder, turmeric, green chillies and ginger.

- Cook on a low heat for 20 minutes, stirring occasionally.

- Add the yoghurt, besan mixture and salt. Cook for 5 minutes.

- Garnish the okra with the coriander leaves. Serve hot.

Sautéed Karela

(Sautéed Bitter Gourd)

Serves 4

Ingredients

4 medium-sized bitter gourds*

Salt to taste

1½ tbsp refined vegetable oil

½ tsp mustard seeds

½ tsp turmeric

½ tsp ginger paste

½ tsp garlic paste

2 large onions, finely chopped

½ tsp chilli powder

¾ tsp jaggery*, grated

Method

- Peel the bitter gourds and slit into halves, lengthways. Discard the seeds and thinly slice each half. Add the salt and set aside for 20 minutes. Squeeze out the water. Set aside again.
- Heat the oil in a saucepan. Add the mustard seeds. Let them splutter for 15 seconds.
- Add the remaining ingredients and fry them on a medium heat for 2-3 minutes. Add the bitter gourd. Mix well. Cook for 5 minutes on a low heat. Serve hot.

Cabbage with Peas

Serves 4

Ingredients

1 tbsp refined vegetable oil

1 tsp mustard seeds

2 green chillies, slit lengthways

¼ tsp turmeric

400g/14oz cabbage, finely shredded

125g/4½oz fresh peas

Salt to taste

2 tbsp desiccated coconut

Method

- Heat the oil in a saucepan. Add the mustard seeds and green chillies. Let them splutter for 15 seconds.
- Add the remaining ingredients, except the coconut. Cook on a low heat for 10 minutes.
- Add the coconut. Mix well. Serve hot.

Potatoes in Tomato Sauce

Serves 4

Ingredients

2 tbsp refined vegetable oil

1 tsp cumin seeds

Pinch of asafoetida

½ tsp turmeric

4 large potatoes, boiled and diced

4 tomatoes, finely chopped

1 tsp chilli powder

Salt to taste

1 tbsp coriander leaves, chopped

Method

- Heat the oil in a saucepan. Add the cumin seeds, asafoetida and turmeric. Let them splutter for 15 seconds.
- Add the remaining ingredients, except the coriander leaves. Mix well. Cook on a low heat for 10 minutes. Garnish with the coriander leaves. Serve hot.

Matar Palak

(Peas and Spinach)

Serves 4

Ingredients

400g/14oz spinach, steamed and chopped

2 green chillies

4-5 tbsp refined vegetable oil

1 tsp cumin seeds

1 pinch of asafoetida

1 tsp turmeric

1 large onion, finely chopped

1 tomato, finely chopped

1 large potato, diced

Salt to taste

200g/7oz green peas

Method

- Grind together the spinach and chillies to a fine paste. Set aside.
- Heat the oil in a saucepan. Add the cumin seeds, asafoetida and turmeric. Let them splutter for 15 seconds.
- Add the onion. Fry on a medium heat till it turns translucent.
- Add the remaining ingredients. Mix well. Cook on a low heat for 7-8 minutes, stirring occasionally.
- Add the spinach paste. Simmer for 5 minutes. Serve hot.

Masala Cabbage

(Spicy Cabbage)

Serves 4

Ingredients

3 tbsp refined vegetable oil

1 tsp cumin seeds

¼ tsp turmeric

1 tsp garlic paste

1 tsp ginger paste

1 large onion, finely chopped

1 tomato, finely chopped

½ tsp chilli powder

Salt to taste

400g/14oz cabbage, finely chopped

Method

- Heat the oil in a saucepan. Add the cumin seeds and turmeric. Let them splutter for 15 seconds. Add the garlic paste, ginger paste and onion. Fry on a medium heat for 2-3 minutes.
- Add the tomato, chilli powder, salt and cabbage. Mix well. Cover with a lid and cook on a low heat for 10-15 minutes. Serve hot.

Aubergine Curry

Serves 4

Ingredients

4 green chillies

2.5cm/1in root ginger

50g/1¾oz coriander leaves, chopped

3 tbsp refined vegetable oil

1 tsp mung dhal*

1 tsp urad dhal*

1 tsp cumin seeds

½ tsp mustard seeds

500g/1lb 2oz small aubergines, chopped into 5cm/2in pieces

½ tsp turmeric

1 tsp tamarind paste

Salt to taste

250ml/8fl oz water

Method

- Grind together the green chillies, ginger and coriander leaves. Set aside.
- Heat the oil in a saucepan. Add the mung dhal, urad dhal, cumin seeds and mustard seeds. Let them splutter for 20 seconds.
- Add the remaining ingredients and the chilli-ginger paste. Mix well. Cover with a lid and simmer for 10 minutes, stirring occasionally. Serve hot.

Simla Mirch ka Bharta

(Spicy Peppers)

Serves 4

Ingredients

3 medium-sized green peppers

3 medium-sized red peppers

3 tbsp refined vegetable oil

2 large onions, finely chopped

6 garlic cloves, finely chopped

2.5cm/1in root ginger, finely chopped

½ tsp chilli powder

¼ tsp turmeric

2 tomatoes, chopped

1 tsp salt

1 tbsp coriander leaves, chopped

Method

- Grill the green and red peppers for 5-6 minutes. Turn frequently to ensure that they are evenly grilled.
- Peel the charred skin, remove the stalks and seeds and chop the peppers into small pieces. Set aside.
- Heat the oil in a saucepan. Add the onions, garlic and ginger. Fry them on a medium heat till the onions are brown.
- Add the chilli powder, turmeric, tomatoes and salt. Sauté the mixture for 4-5 minutes.
- Add the peppers. Mix well. Cover with a lid and cook on a low heat for 30 minutes.
- Garnish the vegetables with the coriander leaves. Serve hot.

Quick Bottle Gourd Curry

Serves 4

Ingredients

1 medium-sized bottle gourd*, peeled and chopped

1 large onion, finely chopped

60g/2oz tomatoes, finely chopped

4-5 garlic cloves, chopped

1 tbsp ketchup

1 tbsp dry fenugreek leaves

½ tsp turmeric

¼ tsp freshly ground black pepper

2 tbsp milk

Salt to taste

1 tbsp coriander leaves, chopped

Method

- Cook all the ingredients, except the coriander leaves, in a saucepan on a medium heat for 20 minutes, stirring occasionally. Cover with a lid.
- Stir the mixture thoroughly. Garnish with the coriander leaves. Serve hot.

Kaala Chana Curry

(Black Chickpea Curry)

Serves 4

Ingredients

250g/9oz kaala chana*, soaked overnight

Pinch of bicarbonate of soda

Salt to taste

1 litre/1¾ pints water

1 small onion

2.5cm/1in root ginger

1 tbsp ghee

1 tomato, diced

½ tsp turmeric

½ tsp chilli powder

8-10 curry leaves

1 tbsp tamarind paste

Method

- Mix the chana with the bicarbonate of soda, salt and half the water. Cook in a saucepan on a medium heat for 45 minutes. Mash and set aside.
- Grind the onion and ginger to a paste.
- Heat the ghee in a saucepan. Add the onion-ginger paste and fry till it turns brown.
- Add the chana mixture and the remaining ingredients. Mix well. Simmer for 8-10 minutes, stirring occasionally. Serve hot.

Kalina

(Mixed Vegetables in Milk)

Serves 4

Ingredients

750ml/1¼ pints milk

2 unripe bananas, peeled and chopped

250g/9oz bottle gourd*, chopped

100g/3½oz cabbage, grated

2 tomatoes, chopped

1 large green pepper, chopped

1 tsp tamarind paste

1 tsp ground coriander

1 tsp ground cumin

2 tsp chilli powder

2 tsp jaggery*, grated

100g/3½oz coriander leaves, finely chopped

2 tbsp khoya*

Salt to taste

1 tbsp coriander leaves, finely chopped

Method

- Heat the milk in a saucepan on a medium heat till it begins to boil. Add the banana and bottle gourd. Mix well. Cook for 5 minutes.
- Add the remaining ingredients, except the coriander leaves. Mix well. Simmer for 8-10 minutes, stirring frequently.
- Garnish the kalina with the coriander leaves. Serve hot.

Tandoori Cauliflower

Serves 4

Ingredients

1½ tsp chilli powder

1½ tsp garam masala

Juice of 2 lemons

100g/3½oz yoghurt

Black salt to taste

1 kg cauliflower florets

Method

- Mix together all the ingredients, except the cauliflower. Then marinate the cauliflower with this mixture for 4 hours.
- Bake in a pre-heated oven at 200°C (400°F, Gas Mark 6) for 5-7 minutes. Serve hot.

Spicy Kaala Chana

Serves 4

Ingredients

500g/1lb 2oz kaala chana*, soaked overnight

500ml/16fl oz water

Salt to taste

3 tbsp refined vegetable oil

Pinch of asafoetida

½ tsp mustard seeds

1 tsp cumin seeds

2 cloves

1cm/½in cinnamon

¼ tsp turmeric

1 tsp ground coriander

1 tsp ground cumin

½ tsp garam masala

1 tsp tamarind paste

1 tbsp coriander leaves, chopped

Method

- Cook the chana with the water and salt in a saucepan on a medium heat for 20 minutes. Set aside.
- Heat the oil in a saucepan. Add the asafoetida and mustard seeds. Let them splutter for 15 seconds. Add the cooked chana and the remaining ingredients, except the coriander leaves. Simmer for 10-15 minutes.
- Garnish the spicy kaala chana with coriander leaves. Serve hot.

Tur Dhal Kofta

(Split Red Gram Dumplings)

Serves 4

Ingredients

600g/1lb 5oz masoor dhal*, soaked overnight

3 green chillies, finely chopped

3 tbsp coriander leaves, chopped

60g/2oz coconut, grated

3 tbsp cumin seeds

Pinch of asafoetida

Salt to taste

Refined vegetable oil for deep frying

Method

- Wash and grind the dhal coarsely. Knead thoroughly with the remaining ingredients, except the oil, to a soft dough. Divide into walnut-sized balls.
- Heat the oil in a saucepan. Add the balls and deep fry them on a low heat till they turn golden brown. Drain the koftas and serve hot.

Shahi Cauliflower

(Rich Cauliflower)

Serves 4

Ingredients

8 garlic cloves

2.5cm/1in root ginger

½ tsp turmeric

2 large onions, grated

4 tsp poppy seeds

2 tbsp ghee

200g/7oz yoghurt, whisked

5 tomatoes, finely chopped

200g/7oz canned peas

1 tsp sugar

2 tbsp fresh single cream

Salt to taste

250ml/8fl oz water

500g/1lb 2oz cauliflower florets, deep fried

8 small potatoes, deep fried

Method

- Grind together the garlic, ginger, turmeric, onions and poppy seeds to a fine paste. Set aside.
- Heat 1 tbsp ghee in a saucepan. Add the poppy paste. Stir-fry for 5 minutes. Add the remaining ingredients, except the cauliflower and potatoes. Cook on a low heat for 4 minutes.
- Add the cauliflower and potatoes. Simmer for 15 minutes and serve hot.

Okra Gojju

(Okra Compote)

Serves 4

Ingredients

500g/1lb 2oz okra, sliced

Salt to taste

2 tbsp refined vegetable oil plus extra for deep frying

1 tsp mustard seeds

Pinch of asafoetida

200g/7oz yoghurt

250ml/8fl oz water

Method

- Toss the okra with salt. Heat the oil in a saucepan and deep fry the okra on a medium heat till golden brown. Set aside.
- Heat 2 tbsp oil. Add the mustard and asafoetida. Let them splutter for 15 seconds. Add the okra, yoghurt and water. Mix well. Serve hot.

Yam in Green Sauce

Serves 4

Ingredients

300g/10oz yam*, thinly sliced

1 tsp chilli powder

1 tsp amchoor*

½ tsp ground black pepper

Salt to taste

Refined vegetable oil for deep frying

For the sauce:

400g/14oz spinach, chopped

100g/3½oz bottle gourd*, grated

Pinch of bicarbonate of soda

3 green chillies

2 tsp wholemeal flour

Salt to taste

3 tbsp refined vegetable oil

1cm/½in root ginger, julienned

1 small onion, finely chopped

Pinch of ground cinnamon

Pinch of ground cloves

Method

- Toss the yam slices with the chilli powder, amchoor, pepper and salt.
- Heat the oil in a saucepan. Add the yam slices. Deep fry them on a medium heat till they turn golden brown. Drain and set aside.
- For the sauce, mix the spinach, bottle gourd and bicarbonate of soda. Steam (see <u>cooking techniques</u>) the mixture in a steamer on a medium heat for 10 minutes.
- Grind this mixture along with the green chillies, flour and salt to a semi-smooth paste. Set aside.
- Heat the oil in a saucepan. Add the ginger and onion. Fry on a medium heat till the onion is brown. Add the ground cinnamon, ground cloves, and the spinach mixture. Mix well. Cook on a medium heat for 8-10 minutes, stirring occasionally.
- Add the yam to this green sauce. Mix well. Cover with a lid and simmer for 4-5 minutes. Serve hot.

Simla Mirch ki Sabzi

(Dry Green Pepper)

Serves 4

Ingredients

2 tbsp refined vegetable oil

2 large onions, finely chopped

¾ tsp ginger paste

¾ tsp garlic paste

1 tsp ground coriander

¼ tsp turmeric

½ tsp garam masala

½ tsp chilli powder

2 tomatoes, finely chopped

Salt to taste

4 large green peppers, chopped

1 tbsp coriander leaves, finely chopped

Method

- Heat the oil in a saucepan. Add the onions, ginger paste and garlic paste. Fry on a medium heat till the onions are brown.
- Add all the remaining ingredients, except the coriander leaves. Mix well. Stir-fry the mixture on a low heat for 10-15 minutes.
- Garnish with the coriander leaves. Serve hot.

Cauliflower Curry

Serves 4

Ingredients

3 tbsp refined vegetable oil

1 tsp cumin seeds

¼ tsp turmeric

1 tsp ginger paste

1 tsp ground coriander

1 tsp chilli powder

200g/7oz tomato purée

1 tsp powdered sugar

Salt to taste

400g/14oz cauliflower florets

120ml/4fl oz water

Method

- Heat the oil in a saucepan. Add the cumin seeds. Let them splutter for 15 seconds.
- Add the remaining ingredients, except the water. Mix well. Add the water. Cover with a lid and simmer for 12-15 minutes. Serve hot

Haaq

(Spinach Curry)

Serves 4

Ingredients

1cm/½ in root ginger, julienned

1 tsp fennel seeds, crushed

2 tbsp refined vegetable oil

2 dried red chillies

¼ tsp asafoetida

1 green chilli, slit lengthways

Salt to taste

400g/14oz spinach, finely chopped

500ml/16fl oz water

Method

- Dry roast (see <u>cooking techniques</u>) the ginger and fennel seeds. Set aside.
- Heat the oil in a saucepan. Add the red chillies, asafoetida, green chilli and salt. Fry this mixture on a medium heat for 1 minute.
- Add the ginger-fennel seed mixture. Fry for a minute. Add the spinach and water. Cover with a lid and simmer for 8-10 minutes. Serve hot.

Dry Cauliflower

Serves 4

Ingredients

3 tbsp refined vegetable oil

1 tsp cumin seeds

¼ tsp turmeric

2 green chillies, finely chopped

1 tsp ginger paste

½ tsp caster sugar

400g/14oz cauliflower florets

Salt to taste

60ml/2fl oz water

10g/¼oz coriander leaves, chopped

Method

- Heat the oil in a saucepan. Add the cumin seeds. Let them splutter for 15 seconds.
- Add the turmeric, green chillies, ginger paste and caster sugar. Fry on a medium heat for a minute. Add the cauliflower, salt and water. Mix well. Cover with a lid and simmer for 12-15 minutes.
- Garnish with the coriander leaves. Serve hot.

Vegetable Korma

(Mixed Vegetables)

Serves 4

Ingredients

3 tbsp refined vegetable oil

1cm/½in cinnamon

2 cloves

2 green cardamom pods

2 large onions, finely chopped

¼ tsp turmeric

½ tsp ginger paste

½ tsp garlic paste

Salt to taste

300g/10oz mixed frozen vegetables

250ml/8fl oz water

1 tsp poppy seeds

Method

- Heat the oil in a saucepan. Add the cinnamon, cloves and cardamom. Let them splutter for 30 seconds.
- Add the onions, turmeric, ginger paste, garlic paste and salt. Fry the mixture on a medium heat for 2-3 minutes, stirring continuously.
- Add the vegetables and water. Mix well. Cover with a lid and simmer for 5-6 minutes, stirring occasionally.
- Add the poppy seeds. Mix well. Simmer for 2 more minutes. Serve hot.

Fried Aubergine

Serves 4

Ingredients

500g/1lb 2oz aubergine, sliced

4 tbsp refined vegetable oil

For the marinade:

1 tsp chilli powder

½ tsp ground black pepper

½ tsp turmeric

1 tsp amchoor*

Salt to taste

1 tbsp rice flour

Method

- Mix the marinade ingredients together. Marinate the aubergine slices with this mixture for 10 minutes.
- Heat the oil in a frying pan. Add the aubergine slices. Fry them on a low heat for 7 minutes. Flip the slices and fry again for 3 minutes. Serve hot.

Red Tomato Curry

Serves 4

Ingredients

1 tbsp peanuts, dry roasted (see <u>cooking techniques</u>)

1 tbsp cashew nuts, roasted (see <u>cooking techniques</u>)

4 tomatoes, chopped

1 small green pepper, chopped

3 tbsp refined vegetable oil

1 tsp ginger paste

1 tsp garlic paste

1 large onion, chopped

1½ tsp garam masala

¼ tsp turmeric

½ tsp sugar

Salt to taste

Method

- Mix the peanuts and cashew nuts together and grind them. Set aside.
- Grind the tomatoes and green pepper together. Set aside.
- Heat the oil in a frying pan. Add the ginger paste and garlic paste. Fry on a medium heat for a minute. Add the onion, garam masala, turmeric, sugar and salt. Fry the mixture for 2-3 minutes.
- Add the peanut-cashew nut mixture and the tomato-pepper mixture. Mix well. Cover with a lid and simmer for 15 minutes. Serve hot.

Aloo Matar Curry

(Potato and Pea Curry)

Serves 4

Ingredients

1½ tbsp refined vegetable oil

1 tsp cumin seeds

1 large onion, finely chopped

½ tsp turmeric

1 tsp ground coriander

1 tsp ground cumin

1 tsp chilli powder

200g/7oz tomato purée

Salt to taste

2 large potatoes, chopped

400g/14oz peas

120ml/4fl oz water

Method

- Heat the oil in a saucepan. Add the cumin seeds. Let them splutter for 15 seconds. Add the onion. Fry it on a medium heat till it turns brown.
- Add the remaining ingredients. Simmer for 15 minutes. Serve hot.

Badshahi Baingan

(Royal Style Aubergine)

Serves 4

Ingredients

8 small aubergines

Salt to taste

30g/1oz ghee

2 large onions, sliced

1 tbsp cashew nuts

1 tbsp raisins

1 tsp ginger paste

1 tsp garlic paste

1 tsp ground coriander

1 tsp garam masala

¼ tsp turmeric

200g/7oz yoghurt

1 tsp coriander leaves, chopped

Method

- Halve the aubergines lengthways. Rub salt on them and set them aside for 10 minutes. Squeeze out excess moisture and set aside again.
- Heat the ghee in a saucepan. Add the onions, cashew nuts and raisins. Fry them on a medium heat till golden brown. Drain and set aside.
- To the same ghee, add the aubergines and fry them on a medium heat till they are tender. Drain and set aside.
- Add the ginger paste and garlic paste to the same ghee. Fry for a minute. Stir in the remaining ingredients. Cook for 7-8 minutes on a medium heat.
- Add the aubergines. Simmer for 2 minutes. Garnish with the fried onions, cashew nuts and raisins. Serve hot.

Potatoes in Garam Masala

Serves 4

Ingredients

3 tbsp refined vegetable oil

1 large onion, finely chopped

10 garlic cloves, finely chopped

½ tsp turmeric

1 tsp garam masala

Salt to taste

3 large potatoes, boiled and diced

240ml/6fl oz water

Method

- Heat the oil in a saucepan. Add the onion and garlic. Fry for 2 minutes.
- Add the remaining ingredients and mix well. Serve hot.

Tamilian Korma

(Tamil-style Mixed Vegetables)

Serves 4

Ingredients

4 tbsp refined vegetable oil

1 tsp cumin seeds

2 large potatoes, chopped

2 large carrots, chopped

100g/3½oz French beans, chopped

Salt to taste

For the spice mixture:

100g/3½oz fresh coconut, shredded

4 green chillies

100g/3½oz coriander leaves, chopped

1 tsp poppy seeds

1 tsp ginger paste

1 tsp turmeric

Method

- Grind all the spice mixture ingredients to a smooth paste. Set aside.
- Heat the oil. Add the cumin seeds. Let them splutter for 15 seconds.
- Add the remaining ingredients and the ground spice mixture. Cook for 15 minutes on a low heat, stirring occasionally. Serve hot.

Dry Aubergine with Onion & Potato

Serves 4

Ingredients

3 tbsp refined vegetable oil

1 tsp mustard seeds

300g/10oz aubergines, chopped

¼ tsp turmeric

3 small onions, finely chopped

2 large potatoes, boiled and diced

1 tsp chilli powder

1 tsp amchoor*

Salt to taste

Method

- Heat the oil in a saucepan. Add the mustard seeds. Let them splutter for 15 seconds.
- Add the aubergines and turmeric. Fry on a low heat for 10 minutes.
- Add the remaining ingredients. Mix well. Cover with a lid and simmer for 10 minutes. Serve hot.

Koftas Lajawab

(Cheese Dumplings in Sauce)

Serves 4

Ingredients

3 tbsp refined vegetable oil

3 large onions, grated

2.5cm/1in root ginger, ground

3 tomatoes, puréed

1 tsp turmeric

Salt to taste

120ml/4fl oz water

For the koftas:

400g/14oz Cheddar cheese, mashed

250g/9oz cornflour

½ tsp freshly ground black pepper

1 tsp garam masala

Salt to taste

Refined vegetable oil for deep frying

Method

- Mix all the kofta ingredients, except the oil, together. Divide into walnut-sized balls. Heat the oil in a saucepan. Add the koftas. Deep fry them on a medium heat till they turn golden brown. Drain and set aside.
- Heat 3 tbsp oil in a saucepan. Add the onions and fry till brown.
- Add the remaining ingredients and mix thoroughly. Cook for 8 minutes, stirring occasionally. Add the koftas to this sauce and serve hot.

Teekha Baingan Masala

(Hot Aubergine)

Serves 4

Ingredients

2 tbsp refined vegetable oil

3 large onions, ground

10 garlic cloves, crushed

2.5cm/1in root ginger, grated

1 tsp tamarind paste

2 tbsp garam masala

Salt to taste

500g/1lb 2oz small aubergines, chopped

Method

- Heat 2 tbsp oil in a saucepan. Add the onions. Fry on a medium heat for 3 minutes. Add the garlic, ginger, tamarind, garam masala and salt. Mix well.
- Add the aubergines. Mix well. Cover with a lid and cook on a low heat for 15 minutes, stirring occasionally. Serve hot.

Vegetable Kofta

(Vegetable Dumplings in Creamy Sauce)

Serves 4

Ingredients

6 large potatoes, peeled and chopped

3 large carrots, peeled and chopped

Salt to taste

Flour for coating

2 tbsp refined vegetable oil plus extra for deep frying

3 large onions, finely sliced

4 garlic cloves, finely chopped

2.5cm/1in root ginger, finely chopped

4 cloves, ground

½ tsp turmeric

2 tomatoes, puréed

1 tsp chilli powder

4 tbsp double cream

25g/scant 1oz coriander leaves, chopped

Method

- Boil the potatoes and carrots in salted water for 15 minutes. Drain and reserve the stock. Add salt to the vegetables and mash them.
- Divide the mash into lemon-sized balls. Coat with the flour and deep fry the koftas in the oil on a medium heat till golden brown. Set aside.
- Heat 2 tbsp of the oil in a saucepan. Add the onions, garlic, ginger, cloves and turmeric. Fry on a medium heat for 4-5 minutes. Add the tomatoes, chilli powder and the vegetable stock. Simmer for 4 minutes.
- Add the koftas. Garnish with the cream and coriander leaves. Serve hot.

Dry Pumpkin

Serves 4

Ingredients

3 tbsp refined vegetable oil

1 tsp cumin seeds

¼ tsp turmeric

¾ tsp ground coriander

Salt to taste

750g/1lb 10oz pumpkin, chopped

60ml/2fl oz water

Method

- Heat the oil in a saucepan. Add the cumin seeds and turmeric. Let them splutter for 15 seconds.
- Add the remaining ingredients. Mix well. Cover with a lid and simmer for 15 minutes. Serve hot.

Mixed Vegetables with Fenugreek

Serves 4

Ingredients

4-5 tbsp refined vegetable oil

1 tsp mustard seeds

½ tsp fenugreek seeds

2 large onions, finely chopped

2 large sweet potatoes, diced

4 small aubergines, diced

2 large green peppers, diced

3 large potatoes, diced

100g/3½oz French beans, chopped

½ tsp turmeric

1 tsp chilli powder

2 tbsp tamarind paste

1 tbsp coriander leaves, chopped

8-10 curry leaves

1 tsp sugar

Salt to taste

750ml/1¼ pints water

Method
- Heat the oil in a saucepan. Add the mustard and fenugreek seeds. Let them splutter for 15 seconds. Add the onions. Fry till translucent.
- Add the remaining ingredients, except the water. Mix well. Add the water. Simmer for 20 minutes. Serve hot.

Dum Gobhi

(Slow Cooked Cauliflower)

Serves 4

Ingredients

2.5cm/1in root ginger, julienned

2 tomatoes, finely chopped

¼ tsp turmeric

1 tbsp yoghurt

½ tsp garam masala

Salt to taste

800g/1¾lb cauliflower florets

Method

- Mix together all the ingredients, except the cauliflower florets.
- Place the cauliflower florets in a saucepan and pour this mixture over it. Cover with a lid and simmer for 20 minutes, stirring occasionally. Serve hot.

Chhole

(Chickpea Curry)

Serves 5

Ingredients

375g/13oz chickpeas, soaked overnight

1 litre/1¾ pints water

Salt to taste

1 tomato, finely chopped

3 small onions, finely chopped

1½ tbsp coriander leaves, finely chopped

2 tbsp refined vegetable oil

1 tsp cumin seeds

1 tsp ginger paste

1 tsp garlic paste

2 bay leaves

1 tsp sugar

1 tsp chilli powder

½ tsp turmeric

1 tbsp ghee

4 green chillies, slit lengthways

½ tsp ground cinnamon

½ tsp ground clove

Juice of 1 lemon

Method

- Mix the chickpeas with half the water and the salt. Cook this mixture in a saucepan on a medium heat for 30 minutes. Remove from the heat and drain the chickpeas.
- Grind 2 tbsp of the chickpeas with half of the tomato, one onion and half the coriander leaves to a fine paste. Set aside.
- Heat the oil in a large saucepan. Add the cumin seeds. Let them splutter for 15 seconds.
- Add the remaining onions, the ginger paste and the garlic paste. Fry this mixture on a medium heat till the onions are brown.
- Add the remaining tomato along with the bay leaves, sugar, chilli powder, turmeric and the chickpea-tomato paste. Fry this mixture on a medium heat for 2-3 minutes.
- Add the remaining chickpeas with the remaining water. Simmer for 8-10 minutes. Set aside.
- Heat the ghee in a small saucepan. Add the green chillies, ground cinnamon and clove. Let them splutter for 30 seconds. Pour this mixture over the chickpeas. Mix well. Sprinkle the lemon juice and the remaining coriander leaves on top of the chhole. Serve hot.

Aubergine Curry with Onion & Potato

Serves 4

Ingredients

3 tbsp refined vegetable oil

2 large onions, finely chopped

1 tsp ginger paste

1 tsp garlic paste

1 tsp ground coriander

1 tsp ground cumin

1 tsp chilli powder

¼ tsp turmeric

120ml/4fl oz water

Salt to taste

250g/9oz small aubergines

250g/9oz baby potatoes, halved

50g/1¾oz coriander leaves, finely chopped

Method
- Heat the oil in a saucepan. Add the onions. Fry till they turn translucent.
- Add the remaining ingredients, except the coriander leaves. Mix well. Simmer for 15 minutes.
- Garnish with the coriander leaves. Serve hot.

Simple Bottle Gourd

Serves 4

Ingredients

½ tbsp ghee

1 tsp cumin seeds

2 green chillies, slit lengthways

750g/1lb 10oz bottle gourd*, chopped

Salt to taste

120ml/4fl oz milk

1 tbsp desiccated coconut

10g/¼oz coriander leaves, finely chopped

Method

- Heat the ghee in a saucepan. Add the cumin seeds and green chillies. Let them splutter for 15 seconds.
- Add the bottle gourd, salt and milk. Simmer for 10-12 minutes.
- Add the remaining ingredients. Mix well. Serve hot.

Mixed Vegetable Curry

Serves 4

Ingredients

3 tbsp refined vegetable oil

1 tsp cumin seeds

1 tsp ground coriander

½ tsp ground cumin

1 tsp chilli powder

¼ tsp turmeric

½ tsp sugar

1 carrot, chopped into strips

1 large potato, diced

200g/7oz French beans, chopped

50g/1¾oz cauliflower florets

Salt to taste

200g/7oz tomato purée

120ml/4fl oz water

10g/¼oz coriander leaves, finely chopped

Method

- Heat the oil in a saucepan. Add the cumin seeds, ground coriander and ground cumin. Let them splutter for 15 seconds.
- Add the remaining ingredients, except the coriander leaves. Mix thoroughly. Simmer for 15 minutes.
- Garnish the curry with the coriander leaves. Serve hot.

Dry Mixed Vegetables

Serves 4

Ingredients

3 tbsp refined vegetable oil

1 tsp cumin seeds

1 tsp ground coriander

½ tsp ground cumin

¼ tsp turmeric

1 carrot, julienned

1 large potato, diced

200g/7oz French beans, chopped

60g/2oz cauliflower florets

Salt to taste

120ml/4fl oz water

10g/¼oz coriander leaves, chopped

Method

- Heat the oil in a saucepan. Add the cumin seeds. Let them splutter for 15 seconds.
- Add the remaining ingredients, except the coriander leaves. Mix thoroughly and cook for 15 minutes on a low heat.
- Garnish with the coriander leaves and serve hot.

Dry Potatoes & Peas

Serves 4

Ingredients

3 tbsp refined vegetable oil

1 tsp cumin seeds

½ tsp turmeric

1 tsp garam masala

2 large potatoes, boiled and diced

400g/14oz cooked peas

Salt to taste

Method

- Heat the oil in a saucepan. Add the cumin seeds and turmeric. Let them splutter for 15 seconds.
- Add the remaining ingredients. Stir-fry on a medium heat for 5 minutes. Serve hot.

Dhokar Dhalna

(Bengal Gram Curry)

Serves 4

Ingredients

300g/10oz chana dhal*, soaked overnight

2 tbsp mustard oil

1 tsp cumin seeds

Salt to taste

5cm/2in cinnamon

4 green cardamom pods

6 cloves

½ tsp turmeric

½ tsp sugar

250ml/8fl oz water

3 large potatoes, diced and fried

Method

- Grind the chana dhal with enough water to form a smooth paste. Set aside.
- Heat half the oil in a saucepan. Add half the cumin seeds. Let them splutter for 15 seconds. Add the dhal paste and the salt. Fry for 2-3 minutes. Drain and spread on a large plate and allow to set. Chop into 2.5cm/1in pieces. Set aside.
- Fry these dhal pieces in the remaining oil till golden brown. Set aside.
- In the same oil, add the remaining ingredients, except the potatoes. Cook for 2 minutes. Add the potatoes and the dhal pieces. Mix well. Cook on a low heat for 4-5 minutes. Serve hot.

Spicy Fried Potatoes

Serves 4

Ingredients

250ml/8fl oz refined vegetable oil

3 large potatoes, chopped into thin strips

½ tsp chilli powder

1 tsp freshly ground black pepper

Salt to taste

Method

- Heat the oil in a saucepan. Add the potato strips. Deep fry them on a medium heat till they turn golden brown.
- Drain and toss well with the remaining ingredients. Serve hot.

www.ingramcontent.com/pod-product-compliance
Lightning Source LLC
Chambersburg PA
CBHW071820080526
44589CB00012B/861